BS/MD Programs— The Complete Guide

2013 EDITION

2013 EDITION
BS/MD Programs— The Complete Guide

GETTING INTO MEDICAL SCHOOL FROM HIGH SCHOOL

EXPANDED AND UP TO DATE

TODD A. JOHNSON

College Admissions Partners • Minnetonka, Minnesota

BS/MD Programs—The Complete Guide:
Getting into Medical School from High School

2013 Edition

by Todd A. Johnson

Published by College Admissions Partners
601 Carlson Parkway Suite 1050
Minnetonka MN 55305
www.collegeadmissionspartners.com
todd@collegeadmissionspartners.com
952-449-5245

ISBN: 978-0-9832132-4-6 trade paperback
        978-0-9832132-5-3 e-book
ISSN: 2168-913X

Manufactured in the United States of America

Design and composition: www.dmargulis.com

To Susie, Kelley and Caitlin,
for all of their support through the years.

Contents

Why I Wrote This Book

Every day, thousands of students dream of one day becoming a doctor. For most of these students, the pathway to medical school involves hard work in high school, so they can get into a good college. Once in college they must work hard to get good grades and eventually study for, and take, the Medical College Admission Test, the MCAT. Despite all of that hard work, many students will not be accepted into a medical school.

But, for the strongest and most dedicated students, for those students who have dreamed of becoming a doctor as long as they can remember, there is another option: early acceptance medical programs (EAMPs), commonly known as BS/MD programs. The EAMPs allow talented students to combine college and medical school into a guaranteed program leading to a medical degree.

Until now, there has been limited information available to students seeking admission to these EAMPs. Students had to search for scattered bits of available information—and much of that information is incorrect.

I wrote this book to help students interested in EAMPs to understand all aspects of the available programs, including what it takes to be a serious candidate for admission. This book provides current information about which programs are available and the criteria needed for admission into the various programs. A website with up-to-date information about BS/MD programs is available at www .collegeadmissionspartners.com.

But, you want to know the details, so let's jump in.

1

What Are
Early Acceptance Programs?

EAMPs. Direct medical programs. BA/MD programs. BS/MD programs. BA/DO programs. These are just a few of the names that early acceptance programs go by. Let's explore the similarities and differences between these types of early acceptance programs.

EAMP is a general term used to describe all of the various types of programs. All of the programs have one basic similarity: each program accepts high school students into both an undergraduate college and a medical school. If you maintain a specified grade point average during college, you have a guaranteed admission to medical school.

The only difference between BA/MD and BS/MD programs is the focus at the undergraduate college. A BA degree, or bachelor of arts, is used by colleges that require a broad educational background. As you work toward a BA degree, you typically take classes in a variety of subject areas during your first two years of college. These include science or math, humanities, and social sciences. In addition, many colleges that give a BA degree require that you show a certain level of competency in a foreign language. You concentrate on classes in your major during the last two years of college. The BA degree is by far the most common degree awarded by most colleges, even for science majors.

A BS degree, or bachelor of science, generally has a stronger focus on taking classes surrounding your major all four years of college. Most of these programs have few, if any, requirements for classes outside a specific major. While as a budding science major, you may think that only a BS degree is for you, be aware that most doctors have a BA degree. What degree you get is more a function of your personal desires and what school you attend than whether you will learn what you need to know to get into medical school. Some of the accelerated medical programs give a BS degree because you may only be in the undergraduate college for two or three years. During that time, you need to take primarily science courses since your undergraduate time is limited.

After finishing the undergraduate portion of a program and receiving the BA or BS, you then spend four years at the medical school and upon completion receive an MD or doctor of medicine degree.

To understand the BA/DO programs, we need a quick history lesson. The DO degree, or the doctor of osteopathy, developed in the late 1800s as an alternative to the MD degree. Doctors with a DO degree get basically the same training as MDs but with additional training in manipulation of the bones. At this point all states recognize the MD and DO degree as both qualified to practice medicine. The American Medical Association allows both types of doctors to become members.

The BA/DO programs are at undergraduate colleges associated with an osteopathic medical college. Otherwise, they are the same as the BA/MD programs. There are BS/DO programs just as there are BS/MD programs. This book deals only with those programs associated with medical schools leading to the MD degree, since these are much more common programs.

How Competitive Are These Programs?

The EAMPs are some of the most selective programs in college admissions. The most selective programs admit only one to two percent of the students who apply. Moreover, at the most selective colleges, the qualifications of the accepted students are extremely high. At Northwestern's Honors Program in Medical Education (HPME) the average SAT score for accepted students is close to a 2,300, and most of the students are in the top one percent of their high school classes. Their average SAT Math Level II score is 775 and the average SAT Chemistry subject test is 762.

Even those early acceptance programs that are "less" selective are extremely selective. The least selective programs still have very high average SAT scores and grade point averages. Make no mistake, no one is guaranteed acceptance into one of these programs regardless of their qualifications.

Many of the less selective early acceptance programs are located at public universities. Some of these public programs are available only to students of that state, and even those that are open to students from other states are much more selective for the out-of-state students. When you review the typical qualifications of the applicants for different programs, keep in mind whether the program is at a public or private university. If the program is public and you are out of state for that program, then you must have much higher qualifications to be competitive for admissions.

One last thought to keep in mind: no matter how strong your qualifications there are no guaranteed acceptances into these programs. Having good grades and test scores merely makes you competitive. But, even perfect grades and perfect test scores are not enough for acceptance. There are additional factors discussed later in the book, such as the quality of your essays and your interview, that help the medical schools determine who to admit into the programs.

How Long Do These Programs Last?

The normal length of education to become a doctor is eight years—four years of undergraduate college and four years of medical school. The early acceptance programs all include the standard four years for medical school.

But there is a difference among the programs on the length of the undergraduate education. Most early acceptance undergraduate programs last four years, which is the typical time to get a college degree. Some of these programs are accelerated, however. There are a few programs where you are at the undergraduate college for only two years and some where you are there three years. These accelerated programs grant the BA or BS degree after you have completed a portion of your medical school education. For example, a six-year EAMP will grant you a BS or BA degree after you have completed two years of college and two years of medical school. A seven-year program grants the undergraduate degree after three years of college and one year of medical school.

How Admissions Decisions Are Made

After you apply to an early acceptance program the first review of your qualifications is made by the undergraduate college's admissions department. Because of the high minimum requirements to qualify for these programs, you will probably be accepted into the undergraduate portion of the program. If you are accepted into the undergraduate college, your file is then sent to the medical school admissions committee for review. The medical school will evaluate your file and decide whether they would like to invite you for an interview at the medical school. Only if you are invited to interview will you continue to be considered for the program. The interview process is described in more detail in Chapter 5. The medical school will determine which students to accept after the interviews are completed.

The Advantages of Early Acceptance Programs

There are a number of potential advantages to the student considering an early acceptance program. The obvious advantage is that if you are accepted into an accelerated program, you no longer have to worry about whether you will be accepted into a medical school. You are accepted.

Early acceptance can also ease your anxiety about the need to get very high grades during college. Most of the early acceptance programs specify minimum grades you must get, often a 3.5 GPA, during college. But the required grades are generally less than you would want to get if you had to worry about applying to medical school. This allows you to focus more on actually learning the subjects and less on the grades.

Students often feel they have more options in the types of courses they take during college while in an early acceptance program. Students trying to impress a medical admissions committee might not want to take classes in the humanities or social sciences. Instead they focus on hard science courses. Students involved with early acceptance programs can take the time to explore their interests outside the laboratory and often become better rounded students—and doctors—as a result.

A third potential benefit of many, but not all, of the programs is the waiver of the requirement to take the Medical College Admission Test, the MCAT, before applying to medical school. Most students who take the MCAT spend a great deal of time preparing for the exam. If your program does not require this test, you have more time to be involved in other activities.

However, even if your program does not require early acceptance students to take the MCAT, there may be reasons to consider taking it. Some scholarships are available based on a student's MCAT score, and the failure to have a score will disqualify you from consideration for the scholarship. Certain combined degree programs such as MD/PhD programs also use the MCAT for admissions purposes. Finally, a few residency programs may consider the MCAT scores to determine placement into the residency.

A fourth benefit offered by many early acceptance programs is a range of enrichment activities for students in the program. As an example of these enrichment activities, let's take a look at Brown University's Program in Liberal Medical Education (PLME).

Brown has a Medicine in Action Program that offers undergraduates and medical students the opportunity to observe practicing physicians. Their Foreign Studies Fellowship Program offers students in the PLME program the "opportunity to integrate an international studies experience into their educational plan." This program provides travel grants to PLME students to engage in international health research or clinical projects in developing countries. In addition, Brown has the PLME Senate, a student organization that encourages early professional development among students involved in the program. Most accelerated programs have similar enrichment programs for their students.

A fifth benefit exists for those programs that last less than eight years. Obviously, in the shortened BS/MD programs you will have fewer years of college and medical school. And that means fewer years of education to pay for.

The Disadvantages of Early Acceptance Programs

Despite all of the wonderful advantages associated with the EAMPs, they are not appropriate for all students. There are several potential disadvantages. Some of the early acceptance programs prohibit a student from applying to medical schools other than the one associated with the program. While this may not seem like much of a disadvantage, medical schools have personalities just like colleges. What is an appropriate medical school for one student may not be the most appropriate for another student. By committing to a particular medical school early, you may be sacrificing the option to attend another medical school that may be more appropriate.

A second disadvantage may exist for those programs that are shorter than the traditional four years of college. If you decide at some point during college that medicine is not what you wish to follow as a profession, there can be problems associated with graduation requirements.

However, the biggest potential disadvantage is a practical one. If you are academically competitive for early acceptance programs, you are likely to be a strong candidate for medical school even if you follow the traditional route of four years of college followed by application to medical school. Many of the early acceptance programs exist at colleges that may be weaker academically than you would traditionally consider. If you decide to follow a traditional path to medical school, you will likely attend a more academically competitive college. By attending a more academically competitive college, you will be a stronger candidate for a more competitive medical school. By going to a more competitive medical school, you may be in a better position to get the residency program you desire. The early acceptance programs limit your options. Whether that disadvantage outweighs the numerous advantages is for you to evaluate.

When to Start Preparing for BS/MD Programs

As I explain in Chapter 2, there are many things you have to do to be a competitive candidate for a BS/MD program. The earlier you start preparing, the better. Seventh and eighth grades are not too early to start working on your academic profile. If you are able to take classes like algebra and geometry in these early grades you will be well positioned to take calculus in high school.

Exploring your extracurricular interests may also start at this stage, so that once you advance in high school you will be able to take leadership roles in your chosen activities. Volunteer efforts can also start at this stage. The strongest candidates will have several years of volunteer time at a single location rather than a smattering of volunteer activities here and there.

Early Medical School Acceptance during College

Some colleges have programs that are named early acceptance programs but they are not the type of early acceptance
being discussed by this book. These alternative early acceptance programs, commonly known as early assurance programs, allow students who are freshmen or sophomores at
a particular college to apply to a program that allows early
acceptance to an associated medical school if all of the required steps of the program are followed. These programs
almost always require the student to take the MCAT and receive a certain minimum score to be admitted to the medical
school. Because these programs do not provide early acceptance into the medical school as a high school student, I will
not spend much time discussing them. However, they may be
appropriate for some students. If you are not accepted into a
true early acceptance program, you may wish to investigate
the possibility of one of these programs as an alternative.

Chapter 2

What It Takes to Be Competitive for BS/MD Programs

The first question I am often asked is this: What does it take to be accepted into one of these EAMPs? Although there is nothing that will guarantee acceptance into an early acceptance program, there are a number of factors that the programs look at in determining who to admit. This chapter will help you understand each of these factors and guide you in the quest to become the strongest possible candidate for an early acceptance program.

First, let's discuss the two factors that are required by many programs to even be considered: grades and test scores.

Grades

The most important factors for admission to an EAMP are your grades and, for some programs, your class rank. The most common requirement is that you be in the top ten percent of your class to be a candidate for an early acceptance program. A few programs require you to be in the top five percent of your class. Some programs have, as an alternative requirement, that you have a certain grade point average to be considered for the program. A minimum 3.8 unweighted GPA is typical.

What happens if a program has a requirement that you be in the top ten percent of your class but your high school does not rank students? In my experience most early acceptance programs will ask for a minimum GPA under these circumstances, so as to not exclude students coming from high schools that don't rank.

A few early acceptance programs have no minimum GPA or class rank requirement for a student to be considered. These programs, however, tend to be the most selective programs. They have no minimum requirement because they don't want to exclude anyone from possible consideration. Don't be misled into thinking that you do not need high grades and class rank just because a program lists no minimums.

The range of grades that make you competitive for these programs varies. However, the minimum is generally an unweighted GPA of 3.5, and that is for state university programs that are seeking to encourage in-state students to apply for a program. To be the most competitive at the majority of the programs, you will need an unweighted GPA of 3.9 or higher and a class rank, if available, in the top one or two percent of your class.

Classes

Closely related to your grades are the classes you take to get those grades. BS/MD programs like to see students who have challenged themselves in their classes. Ideally, students will take four years of each of the five core subjects: math, science, English, social studies, and a single foreign language. While few colleges require this type of program, most of the students that you will competing against will have most, if not all, of these classes.

Some BS/MD programs have specific requirements on which classes students must take to be able to apply. Most commonly they require a year each of biology, chemistry, and physics; but many colleges also require four years of English and four years of math. And while few colleges require calculus, I cannot recall any of my students getting admitted to a BS/MD program without having calculus. Whether it is

AB or BC doesn't seem to make any difference as long as you have one of those courses or the equivalent.

So, besides asking that you take all of the core subjects, what do BS/MD programs mean when they talk about challenging classes. Usually it means that students will have taken an appropriate number of AP or IB classes, particularly in the sciences and math. While you don't need to take every AP class your school offers, you do need to take a significant number. My typical BS/MD students have taken between six and eight AP classes while in high school.

I am sometimes asked if it makes any difference if a student takes AP classes versus IB classes. I have not seen any difference in admissions rates for one program versus the other. I can say that admissions officers are impressed with students taking IB classes who get a full IB diploma.

Test Scores

The second factor required for early acceptance programs is a strong standardized test score. Most programs require a minimum SAT score between 1,350 and 1,450 exclusive of the writing sub-score. Again, these are minimum requirements. To be the most competitive you should have the highest test score possible.

While the majority of colleges super-score the SAT for general admissions, early acceptance programs do not typically super-score the SAT for admissions to these programs. (Super-scoring means taking the highest subsection score from multiple test dates and combining the highest scores to make a super-score. For example, suppose you take the SAT twice and the first time receive a 600 verbal and 700 math. The second time you take the SAT you receive a 700 verbal and 620 math. Although the highest score from one sitting is the 1,320 from the second test, a college that super-scores will combine the 700 verbal from the second test with the 700 math from the first test to give a super-score of 1,400.)

Some programs also state a minimum ACT score for students taking that test. Most commonly, the minimum ACT score is a 30 composite score. Those programs that don't state a minimum ACT convert an ACT score into an SAT score. A few programs prefer to see either the SAT or the ACT test, and they will tell you their preference.

In addition to the SAT or ACT tests, many of the programs also want to see two SAT subject test scores. Some programs tell you specifically what subject test scores they would like to see; but if they don't say, the best option is to take the Math II subject test and either the Chemistry or the Biology subject test. Again, to be most competitive you want to score greater than 700 on each of the subject tests.

All right, you say you have great grades and your tests scores are wonderful. So what are some of the other factors considered for admissions into early acceptance programs?

Research Experience

Most competitive students applying to early acceptance programs have some type of scientific research experience, most commonly in biology or chemistry. This is often as a result of a research opportunity at a university that the student participated in during one of their summers but may also have occurred during the school year. While there are no specific requirements that an applicant have research experience, the early acceptance programs look very favorably on this type of experience, as it further confirms your interest in a scientific field. Contrary to what many people may think, this research does not need to be related to a medical field.

A common question I am asked is, How does a student find a research opportunity? There are two basic ways this occurs. The first option, which I prefer, is to have a student find their own research at a college or university that is close to where they live. They can often do this by investigating the professors at the university to see who is doing research that the student finds interesting. The student can then contact the professor and ask to be part of the research team, usually during the summer before junior year or summer before senior year. To have the best chance of having a professor agree to this, you will need to make it clear that you are interested in research and that you are a strong student in math and science. You should first contact the professor in the January before the summer you wish to do the research.

The second option to get research is usually simpler. There are many colleges around the country that sponsor summer research opportunities for high school students. Some of them are competitive and require an application, and these generally are available in January and February. These programs also charge for the student to participate, and they can be quite expensive.

The reason I prefer the first option, aside from the obvious cost savings, is that it shows a certain level of maturity for a student to contact a college professor and arrange their own research opportunity. And as we will see later in this chapter, maturity is a factor in admissions for BS/MD programs.

Volunteer Activities

Most colleges like to see applicants who have volunteered their time to help others. This is particular true for early acceptance programs, because they are looking for students who show compassion. There are few better ways to show compassion than by volunteering. Ideally, some of this volunteer effort should occur in a health-related setting such as a clinic, hospital, or nursing home.

There is no minimum number of volunteer hours needed, and it is not necessary to record the number of hours you have as a volunteer. However, it is obvious to anyone if you have not been serious about showing true compassion. This is not about fulfilling a requirement. This is about really showing that you care. I generally advise students that the longer a particular volunteer effort has been going on, the greater the weight it will be given. Ideally, you will have volunteered for more than one year at one or more facilities. You do not need to devote all of your time to volunteering. One or two hours a week, if done consistently during the year, is sufficient.

Physician Shadowing

Early acceptance programs also like to see that a student has performed some type of physician shadowing, ideally with more than one physician. Early acceptance programs want to admit only those students who are truly committed to becoming a physician. Many students start college declaring their intent to become physicians; yet the majority of these students drop out along the way for various reasons. Early acceptance programs want to minimize the number of students who change their minds about becoming physicians. One of the ways you can convince the programs you are serious about becoming a physician is to show that you have followed one or more doctors around to see what their typical day is like.

Many doctors are happy to have a student shadow them if you explain that you are committed to attending medical school and want to experience what their actual work is like. Many students follow a doctor around in a clinical setting, but many also are able to make hospital rounds and even observe surgery. It does not matter what type of physician you shadow; but if you think you might have a particular interest in one field of medicine, then see if you can shadow a physician who specializes in that field. There is no minimum amount of time you have to do the shadowing, but I usually recommend that students try to spend at least 40 hours shadowing a physician. If you wish to do more than this, it is fine; but volunteering is usually a better way to spend your time after 40 hours.

Extracurricular Activities

Another significant factor in the admissions process for early acceptance programs is the evaluation of the student's extra-curricular activities.

There should be a focus on leadership in your activities during the junior and senior year. Early acceptance programs are not interested in students who join many different activ-ities but do not seriously pursue any of them. Rather, a long-term commitment to the activity is what these programs are looking for. Ideally, you should be involved in those activities that interest you the most; and it is best if you have some leadership experience in those activities.

People often ask what the best extracurricular activity is, but the reality is that there is no one right activity. Col-leges want to see you involved in activities that are of par-ticular interest to you. These may be activities related to school, but they can just as easily be activities outside of school. The focus of these activities, however, is often differ-ent for early acceptance students than for students applying only to highly selective colleges.

The most selective colleges are looking for students who are specialists in a particular activity. These are the stu-dents who have focused all of their interest on a select few activities—the student whose life revolves around the clari-net, the stage, or the chemistry lab.

Early acceptance programs, on the other hand, tend to favor students who have a somewhat broader background. You might be involved in the band, student government, and science Olympiad all at the same time. As long as you have been seriously involved in each of your activities, you will be a strong candidate. What does it mean to be seriously involved? It means that you have been involved with the activity through most, if not all, of your high school career, devoting substantial time to the activity and resulting in a leadership position of some sort.

One difference with the extracurricular activities for those students interested in early acceptance programs is the focus on health-related activities. This might include involvement in, or the founding of, a chapter of Future Doctors of America, involvement with science Olympiad, or other activities that have some relationship with the health care field.

Another way in which the focus of extracurricular activities differs for early acceptance programs is the focus on volunteer effort. While all highly selective colleges like to see students who have a compassionate side, this is particularly important for students applying to early acceptance programs. Being a physician will pay well, but there is also a huge commitment to caring for others that is needed to be a good physician. Medical schools, and early acceptance programs in particular, are not looking for the student whose sole goal in becoming a doctor is to make lots of money. They are seeking the student for whom the practice of medicine is a passion. Substantial volunteer effort is a great way to show the medical school that you have the compassion needed to be a great physician.

Early acceptance programs like all volunteer activity, but they particularly like to see involvement in volunteer activities that are health-related. I have had many students who volunteered in nursing homes. Nursing homes are often a good place to volunteer, because they don't typically have many restrictions on who can volunteer or what they do. Some of my students have gone to the nursing homes on a regular basis to visit with residents of the home. Others went to play musical instruments, read books to those who are vision-impaired, or help with feeding residents.

Nursing homes are not the only place you can volunteer. Many hospitals will gladly work with a student who wishes to volunteer. This often involves helping in a gift shop or helping direct people who are visiting the hospital. While this type of volunteering is good, it is best if you can be in a position of interacting with patients. For instance, a few students of mine have had the opportunity to volunteer in an emergency room or an outpatient surgery area. This type of volunteering, however, can be hard to come by in a hospital. That is why the nursing home setting can be more useful.

Many students, in completing the list of extracurricular activities on the application, want to list every activity they have been involved in since they were young. This is not a good idea. You want to focus your extracurricular activities on those that show your interest in health care, that high-light your leadership, or that reflect those activities that you have been seriously involved with. That one hour that you rang the bell for the Salvation Army should not be listed. Although it is a volunteer activity, listing this type of limited involvement activity either looks like you don't have enough serious volunteer activities or you are shallow and pander-ing. Neither is the impression you want to give a medical school admissions committee.

There are two basic ways to provide the colleges with information about your extracurricular activities. The most common is through the activity list of the Common Applica-tion. The Common Application provides room for ten activi-ties. For each activity you can list the years devoted to the activity, the number of hours per week, the number of weeks per year, your position in the activity, and a brief statement of what the activity involves. You can also indicate if this is an activity that you intend to continue in college.

There are several advantages to using the activity list of the Common Application as your only list of activities. First, it is simple. You don't have to worry about how to structure a list of activities; the list is ready for you to complete. And because of the limited space available, you have to choose only those activities that are most important to you and to be succinct in describing each activity.

The second advantage is that the activity list on the Common Application makes it simple for the college admissions reader to review all of your activities at a glance. Given that a typical application only gets fifteen to twenty minutes of review for the entire application, having a convenient list of the most important activities is helpful. For most students I recommend that they use the Common Application list for activities as their exclusive list.

However, there is another option that is appropriate for some students. For some students with a large number of strong activities, the supplemental activities résumé may be appropriate. This supplemental résumé is a replacement for the activities list on the Common Application. The major advantage of the supplemental résumé is that it lets you provide greater detail about specific activities and it allows the listing of a greater number of activities. Many counselors encourage all of their students to submit a supplemental résumé rather than use the application list of the Common Application. While this may seem like a wise idea, I believe that it actually works to the disadvantage of many students.

There are several issues that should be considered by the student who is considering using a supplemental résumé. First, remember that a college admissions officer has limited time to look at the entire application. As I mentioned earlier, fifteen to twenty minutes is typical for the time to review an application.

Now imagine that you have just submitted a three-page résumé of activities. If the admissions officer looks at your entire résumé, they will have that much less time to review the rest of your application, including your grades, classes, test scores, and essays. What typically happens in these situations is that the admissions officer spends the usual amount of time looking at your grades, classes, test scores, and essays. They then take the limited amount of time they have left to scan over your résumé. If the résumé is too detailed, or too long, the admissions officer may miss some of your activities just because they don't have time to review each application in that kind of detail. You may also annoy the admissions reader because they are trying to be fair to everyone whose application they have to read. If they feel that they have to spend more time on your résumé than on some other student's, it will generally not help, and may hurt, your chance of admissions.

The second factor to consider if you are thinking about doing a supplemental résumé is whether you really have enough activities to justify such a résumé. There are some students that have an incredible amount of serious extracurricular activities that cannot be accounted for by the Common Application. But this is the unusual circumstance.

The third factor to consider is how it looks on your application that you are not able to write succinctly to describe your activities. Colleges using the Common Application do so intentionally to make sure that they get the information they require. Colleges are not pushing the Common Application to increase the number of listings for activities or to give more space for the description of the activities. That is because they know that for most students, the allowed space is sufficient to list the most important activities.

If you really believe you have too many activities for the Common Application, or that you need to provide more detail on your activities than the space on the Common Application allows, try to limit the supplemental résumé to one page of single spaced type. Follow the same format as the Common Application so that similar information is included in your supplemental résumé. Choose an ordinary serif typeface that is easily read on paper or computer monitor, such as Century Schoolbook (what you are reading now) or Garamond, in 12-point size. If space is tight, you can use Times New Roman, instead. Do not try to demonstrate your creativity by selecting a script font or an informal font such as

Comic Sans. Doing so will detract from the image you are presenting.

Remember that the Common Application provides a Short Answer Essay that allows you to "elaborate on one of your activities (extracurricular, personal activities, or work experience)." If you just have one activity that needs more information than you can provide on the Common Application activity list, provide that information in this essay rather than using a supplemental résumé.

Finally, the Common Application also provides a space for you to provide any additional information that you would like the college to know about. This is another space that can be used to expand on your activities without using a supplemental résumé. As of the writing of this book, there is some question on whether the Common Application will continue to have space for additional information. If this is eliminate, your only option to submit a résumé would be as an additional document.

Recommendations

Most EAMPs require two teacher recommendations and a counselor recommendation. For most colleges, recommendations have little influence on the admissions decisions. However, in programs that are extremely competitive, such as EAMPs, any small advantage should be used.

To get the best recommendations from your teachers and counselor you want to make sure that they have information on all of your background. One easy way is to provide them with a résumé. Remember that résumé you wanted to put together for the application? Use that résumé instead to provide complete information to your recommenders.

Ideally, the recommendation will focus on those issues that are important to an EAMP. Comments about your maturity, your helpfulness in the classroom, your volunteer activities, and your leadership are all helpful. You want to be sure that your recommender is aware of your commitment to attending medical school, and you may ask them to comment on this focus. Familiarity of the recommender with any extended health care volunteer activities would also be helpful.

Students often do not have a strong relationship with their high school counselor because the counselor has a large number of students to work with. If that is true of your counselor, you need to make every effort to get to know your counselor as well as possible before they need to write your recommendation. Colleges understand that high schools often have high counselor-to-student ratios so will not penalize you if you don't get a detailed recommendation from your counselor. But, if you can get a good recommendation from your counselor, it is one more small step in helping the application reader understand who you are.

Students often wish to provide more recommendations than are asked for by the college. It is the rare situation when it is appropriate to send additional recommendation letters. Colleges ask for the information that they think they need to make a reasoned decision. If they wanted more recommendations, they would ask for them. The only time it is appropriate to provide an additional recommendation is if that recommender can offer a perspective on an important aspect of your background that is not addressed elsewhere in the application.

Final Thoughts

Colleges and in particular medical schools are not just looking for the brightest students. Yes, you need the grades and test scores to be eligible to apply to BS/MD programs. But, even the strongest students need to show more to be successful in applying to these programs. You also need to show that you have the passion to be a physician and the compassion to be a good doctor. You need to show that you have the maturity to handle the pressure of medical school and the life of a physician. You must communicate that you are conscientious but also personable.

How do you show that you have these personality characteristics? This information should come out in all aspects of your application. Your college and medical school essays, your activity list, your recommendations, and your interview all are opportunities to communicate who you are beyond your transcript. As you proceed through your application to a BS/MD program do not lose sight of who you are and how you might communicate that to the programs.

Chapter 3

Finding the Right Program

Now that you know what you have to do to be competitive for an EAMP, let's look at the various choices you have to make to ensure you find the right program for your needs.

What Is the Length of the Early Acceptance Program?

As we have already seen, these programs can last six, seven, or eight years. Six-year programs are probably the least common, with eight-year programs the most common. The advantage to the six-year programs is you can finish a traditional eight-year program in only six years. You do this by focusing on the required basic science classes during the first two years of undergraduate education. You then start the medical school portion of your training and are awarded your undergraduate degree after the first two years of medical school.

What you lose from a shortened program is the ability to take classes outside of the basic sciences, since you have only two years of undergraduate education. Doctors need to understand the basic sciences, and all early acceptance programs preserve that need. However, being a doctor involves much more than just understanding the science.

Having a background in the humanities can give a doctor a broader base of knowledge when dealing with patients. The study of subjects such as sociology, psychology, and anthropology may help you understand the patient from a personal standpoint. Having additional years of undergraduate college also allows you to study a foreign language in more detail. Having more years of college also allows students to become better communicators, and being able to talk with patients is a vital part of most physicians' lives.

Does the Program Exempt Students from Taking the MCAT?

The Medical College Admission Test (MCAT) often creates a great deal of anxiety among students interested in attending medical school. At most medical schools, the results of the MCAT is second only to a student's college grades in determining who will be admitted to medical school. The MCAT generally requires a great deal of time and preparation if a student is to score well.

Many of the early acceptance programs do not require that you take the MCAT before starting the medical school portion of your education. The opportunity to avoid the MCAT is a major motivation for many students to consider early acceptance programs. If you are concerned about taking the MCAT, you may want to focus on programs that do not require the submission of the test. Even if you are a strong test taker, you may wish to avoid the MCAT so that you can use the time normally taken in test preparation for other purposes. In fact, avoiding the MCAT could give you enough time to take another class or become more involved in a particular activity.

There are a number of early acceptance programs that require the MCAT. Among those programs, some require a minimum MCAT score and others have no set minimum score. If the program that you are considering is one that requires the MCAT be taken, check to see if there is any required minimum score. If not, much of the pressure associated with the MCAT is reduced even if you need to take the test.

If the program you are interested in has a minimum score, look to see how high that score is. If it is a relatively low score, you may not need to devote a great deal of time to the MCAT. However, some programs have a relatively high minimum MCAT score. The early acceptance program between Lehigh University and Drexel University College of Medicine has a minimum MCAT score of 31. A score of 31 on the MCAT is the average MCAT score of students admitted to the Drexel College of Medicine through the regular admissions route. Thus, at a program like the Lehigh–Drexel program, a student in the early acceptance program would need to study more for the MCAT than would a student applying to Drexel University College of Medicine.

How Clinical Training Is Addressed by the Medical School

The first two years of medical school are typically devoted to an in-depth look at the systems of the body. This is primarily an academic approach in the classroom or the laboratory. In the last two years of medical school, the students go to various clinical sites that allow them to actually start interacting with patients.

There is a current move among some medical schools to better integrate clinical training and classroom training. Some programs provide clinical experiences in the first year, but the extent of early clinical experiences varies by program. If you are interested in having clinical experiences all four years of medical school, you will want to ask the medical school how they handle clinical training.

The other question you should investigate is what clinical options are available during medical school. Ideally, the clinical sites are in large hospitals or clinical settings where you can see a variety of medical problems. The broader the types of patients and problems you see, the more likely you will have the experience to do well on the national medical tests required during medical school. If a clinical setting has little variety in the types of patients seen, you will be at a disadvantage when taking the national exams.

What Is the Medical School's USMLE Pass Rate?

This question is closely related to the one we just discussed regarding the available clinical sites. Medical students must take a series of exams known in general as the United States Medical Licensing Exam. There are several parts to this exam, taken at various times during a medical student's education. Part 1 of the exam is taken after the first two years of medical school. This part of the exam tests your understanding of the basic scientific concepts necessary to practice medicine.

Part 2 of the exam is typically taken during the fourth year of medical school. Part 2 itself is divided into two tests. The first exam of Part 2, CK, tests the clinical knowledge you have acquired. The second part of the exam, CS, tests the clinical skills you have acquired as you near completion of your formal education. It is in Part 2 of the exam that the program's clinical sites can be important.

Obviously, you wish to see pass rates as close to one hundred percent as possible on both portions of this exam for each early acceptance program you are considering. In 2007, the pass rate for Part 1 examinations from students attending a US or Canadian MD program was ninety-three percent. For students attending a DO program, the average pass rate was eighty-one percent.

The pass rate that year for Part 2 CK examinations for students attending a US or Canadian MD program was ninety-four percent. For those students in a DO program, the pass rate was eighty-seven percent. For Part 2 CS exams, the pass rate was ninety-seven percent for US or Canadian MD programs and ninety-three percent for DO programs.

If the program you are considering has pass rates on either section of the USMLE substantially lower than the national average, you should ask pointed questions on why they have a lower pass rate.

How Effective Is the Medical School at Matching Students into One of the Student's Top Three Residency Choices?

Once you finish medical school, the next step in your education is the residency, where you spend several years working on your particular specialty. The process of determining where the residency will occur is known as a match program. Students specify their preferences for where they would like to do their residency, and residency programs then look at the list of students who wish to attend their program to see which students they will accept. There are a variety of factors that go into the decision of who will be offered a residency at a particular program. Common factors include the strength of the medical school, the grades earned by the student, and the scores the student received on their USMLE exam.

As a student, your biggest concern is getting into one of your top options for a residency program. At times, even strong students from strong medical schools will not match one of their top programs. If few of the medical school's students match their top options for a residency program, you will want to ask questions.

What Are the Requirements of the Undergraduate Portion of the Program?

Although each of these programs guarantees admission to a medical school upon completion of the undergraduate study, there are requirements during the undergraduate years that must be met. You need to understand what those requirements are for each of the program you are interested in. Usually you need to maintain a minimum overall grade point average as well as a minimum grade point average for science and math courses. Most commonly this is a 3.5 GPA. Some can be higher. For instance, Washington University's

University Scholar in Medicine program requires that students maintain a 3.8 GPA. If you have a high school GPA of 4.0, you may not think that sounds bad. But be aware that getting a GPA of 3.8 at a competitive college is not as easy as it may sound.

Other common requirements for students in these programs include occasional evaluations of your work by members of the BS/MD committee, attending scheduled meetings related to the program, and participation in volunteer service projects.

What Is the Completion Rate for the Program?

You will want to ask the early acceptance programs how many of the students who start the program actually finish. There are many reasons why someone might decide not to complete an early acceptance program. Some students may decide that their interest in medicine is not as strong as they thought it was before starting the program, while others find that academically, the program is more difficult than they thought. You should not be concerned if a few people leave the program each year.

However, if a large percentage of people leave the program, you need to ask further questions to find out why people are leaving the program. The biggest concern is if people are not finishing the program because they were not able to meet the minimum grade requirements. You should ask how many people leave the program because they were not successful academically. This might be because students did not have adequate preparation in high school, or it may be that there are problems getting the required grades in a required class. The University of Alabama states that fifteen percent of students admitted to their program fail out and fifty percent are on probation at some time during their undergraduate years. You will want to know that same information for the programs you are considering.

What Ability Do You Have to Attend
Other Colleges or Medical Schools?

Just as not all colleges are appropriate for all students, not all medical schools are appropriate for all students. You may find that the focus of the medical school associated with the early acceptance program is not consistent with your focus. Or you may find that the teaching style at the medical school makes it difficult for you to learn the necessary lessons. If you find, for whatever reason, that the medical school just is not appropriate, what opportunities do you have to apply to another medical school?

Most programs specify that you lose your guaranteed spot at the medical school if you decide to apply to other medical schools. You would still have the option to be considered as a regular applicant, but you would have no advantages over other candidates. If you think you may wish to have the option to apply to other medical schools, you should only consider those programs that allow you to maintain your guaranteed spot even while applying to other medical schools.

If you decide that the undergraduate college is not appropriate you will want to know how easy it is to transfer to another college. The sequence of courses with some programs may make it difficult to transfer to another college. This is particularly true for the six- and seven-year accelerated programs. You should ask how many students transfer to another college and, for those that transfer, whether they have any difficulties with the transfer process.

What Happens if You Decide
Not to Attend Medical School

No one goes into an EAMP with the thought they might change their mind and decide not to attend medical school. But, every year, certain students decide that medical school is just not right for them. Even if you are sure that this will never happen to you, it only takes a few questions to find out what will happen if you have a change of heart.

In most programs, deciding not to pursue medical school is not a problem, because you would just continue on as a regular college student at the undergraduate college. However, there can be problems if you are on an accelerated program that lasts six or seven years. Remember that for the accelerated programs, the reduced time is at the undergraduate level. What happens if you are in a six-year program and, in the first year of medical school, you decide medicine just isn't for you? You will not receive your undergraduate degree until you finish your second year of medical school. But, if you don't finish two years of medical school, what do you need to do to finish your undergraduate degree?

Remember that you are choosing not only an undergraduate college but also a medical school when you apply to an early acceptance program. For the best fit you need to make sure you are applying not only to the best college for your needs but also to the best medical school for your needs.

If you have more questions about a particular program, you should talk to people involved in the program, including professors at the undergraduate and medical school level. If there are concerns about the number of people who leave the program, you should ask about this issue. You may also wish to talk with students who are currently in the program to get their thoughts on how well the program is run and whether they feel prepared to advance to the medical school or take the USMLE exams. You should be able to ask the program to give you the contact information for current students who can answer your questions.

Chapter 4

The Application Essays

Most students applying to early acceptance programs are very high achieving students with high grades and high test scores. So how do colleges distinguish between all of these strong students? One way is by reviewing the application essays. In this chapter we will look in more detail at the various essays that may be required in the application for early acceptance programs. First, let's examine the essays required for the undergraduate application.

Undergraduate College Application Essay

Colleges use the undergraduate application essays for several purposes. First, they want to see how well you can write. The ability to write well is critical in college regardless of your major. Reviewing your application essays is one of the ways colleges evaluate your ability to write well. They also look at your grades in English classes and your score on the writing section of the SAT or ACT as further verification of your ability to write.

A second purpose of the application essay is to provide the application reader some insight into the applicant as a person beyond the grades and test scores. We will talk about what to write about in a little bit, but understand for now that you do not want to be discussing grades and test scores in your application essay. This is your chance to showcase something else about why you are a strong applicant.

Most of the early admissions medical programs (EAMPs) use the Common Application for the application to the undergraduate college. The Common Application has several essays that both allow you to show the application reader how well you write and to reveal a little more about the person behind the application.

Before we start talking about the essays, just a few words on the mechanics of writing an essay. You do not need to title your essay unless you think that a title will add something to the essay itself. In most cases, the writing should be able to convey your story without a title. If it does not, then you need to work some more on the essay.

Unless the instructions specifically ask for single line spacing, use double line spacing, with ample page margins, as this improves readability. Use the same typeface and size you chose for the Common Application, such as 12-point Garamond or Century Schoolbook (or another ordinary-looking serif typeface). You want the reader to focus on what you wrote, not on your taste in exotic fonts.

Enough of the mechanics. Let's talk about the essays themselves.

Common Application Essays

The main essay on the Common Application is known as the personal essay. This has a minimum length of 250 words with a maximum length of 650 words. In the past the Common Application has recommended a maximum length of 500 words but has not enforced that limit. Starting with the 2013 application they have indicated that they will enforce a word limit of 650 words.

Be aware, however, that the essay is a very personal piece of writing, and focusing on length can make for a bad essay. I have seen wonderful essays that barely made the 250 word limit. Write to communicate what you wish to communicate, and stop writing. If it is over 650 words, then review the essay to focus on the most important elements while not exceeding 650 words.

Your first job with the personal essay is to decide which prompt you wish to write about. The Common Application has in the past used six standard essay prompts, which are listed here.

1. Evaluate a significant experience, achievement, risk you have taken, or ethical dilemma you have faced and its impact on you.
2. Discuss some issue of personal, local, national, or international concern and its importance to you.
3. Indicate a person who has had a significant influence on you, and describe that influence.
4. Describe a character in fiction, a historical figure, or a creative work (as in art, music, science, etc.) that has had an influence on you, and explain that influence.
5. A range of academic interests, personal perspectives, and life experiences adds much to the educational mix. Given your personal background, describe an experience that illustrates what you would bring to the diversity in a college community, or an encounter that demonstrated the importance of diversity to you.
6. Topic of your choice.

Prompts © The Common Application. Used with permission.

Starting in 2013, the essay prompts will change each year, although the people at the Common Application have said that the essay prompts will be broad in nature to allow students some flexibility on what to write about. You can use the above prompts to give you some idea of the types of questions that might be asked. One choice is not better than another. Read through each of the prompts and see if there is any one that is particularly appealing to you.

In brainstorming for ideas to write about, you want to keep in mind that the application reader is looking for a little insight into who you are beyond grades and test scores. They have your transcript, your official test scores, and a list of activities in the application. Do not repeat any of that information. You want to communicate one small part of who you are or something in your life that has influenced who you are or how you think. The biggest mistake most students make in writing the college application essay is to tackle too broad a topic. The purpose of this book is not to go into great detail about writing the college application. However, because of the importance of the application, I would strongly urge you to consider looking at one of the books that discuss writing the college application essay. One of the best is Harry Bauld's book, *On Writing the College Application Essay.*

While guiding you through the college application essay is not the goal of this book, improving your standing as an applicant to an early admissions medical program is. So how do you write the personal essay to enhance your application to such programs? Always keep in mind what qualities the colleges and medical colleges are looking for in successful applicants. They are looking for a student with a long-standing passion to become a physician. They are looking for students with leadership abilities, with maturity, and with compassion. You may not be able to write an essay that covers each of these topics, but you can focus your essay on one of them. Which one does not matter, although I would lean toward an essay that shows you have true compassion for others.

The Common Application also has a short answer section where the prompt is "Please briefly elaborate on one of your extracurricular activities or work experiences in the space below or on an attached sheet (150 words or fewer)." It does not matter which activity you choose to write about, but it should be one that strengthens your résumé for early acceptance programs. Writing about your involvement with the baseball team may make a good short essay, but something that relates to your involvement with an activity that shows compassion or a health-related activity would be even better.

One additional caution when writing the Common Application essays. While it is fine to be self-assured, you want to make sure that you do not come across as bragging about yourself. Medical schools do not want students who are self-impressed. In your essay don't talk about how everyone looks up to you or how you are well known for your volunteer activities. You want to present a more humble approach in your essays. Let your recommendations talk about what a great student you are that everyone looks up to.

In the past the Common Application provided you with even more room to elaborate on your background and interests in the Additional Information section of the application. This prompt said that you can "Include any additional information that you would like to provide." As of the writing of this book the final decision on whether to keep this section or eliminate it has not been made. If it is available, this is yet another opportunity to communicate your unique strength and why you should be considered a strong candidate for an early acceptance program. You have 2,000 characters in which to provide your response, and this is a fairly significant space. It is usually in your best interest to write something in this section, although you do not need to use the entire 2,000 characters if you can answer in less space. Remember that your entire application will be read in a limited period, so you do not want to waste space.

Thus, the Common Application itself provides two or three different places to discuss some aspect of who you are. Each of the sections should discuss a different aspect of your life. You do not want to talk about the humanitarian club you founded in all three sections, for instance. This makes it sound as if you don't have the depth of involvement to be a serious candidate for early acceptance.

If that was not enough space to talk about yourself and your involvement with different activities, most colleges also have supplemental essays to the Common Application.

Most of the college-specific essays fall into one of two types: "What will you add to our community" questions; and "Why are you interested in our college" questions. Rice University, for instance, asks: "The quality of Rice's academic life and the Residential College System are heavily influenced by the unique life experiences and cultural traditions each student brings. What perspective do you feel that you will contribute to life at Rice?" This question from Rice makes it clear that they are not seeking everyday, boring students. They want students who are interesting and interested in the world around them. If you have health care experiences in a foreign country, this would be a great time to write about that experience. It answers the question about what makes you interesting, and it once again ties in your interest in the health care field.

Northwestern University's essay question focuses more on why you wish to attend that college but again leaves room for you to distinguish yourself from other applicants: "What are the unique qualities of Northwestern— and of the specific undergraduate school to which you are applying— that make you want to attend the University? In what ways do you hope to take advantage of the qualities you have identified?" When answering a question about why you wish to attend a particular college, you should be specific. Look at your answer after you have it written. If you can substitute the name of another college in place of the college you are applying to, the answer is too generic.

Look at the mission statement of each college that asks for an essay like this. The college's mission statement tells you how the college views itself and how they believe that they are different from other colleges. Another idea is to look at the departmental webpage of the major you are considering. Most colleges give biographies of the faculty in that department. If you find a particular professor that is working on something that is of interest to you, reference your interest in that professor's work in your essay.

If you are applying to an EAMP that does not use the Common Application, you may have less work to do for the initial college application. The University of Missouri at Kansas City early acceptance program, for instance, has no essay requirement for the undergraduate application. Some of the other non–Common Application colleges do have essay requirements, but they tend to be fairly general questions that you may be able to use the Common Application personal essay for.

Medical School Essays

You have submitted your undergraduate application; and now, if you are lucky, you will be asked to answer some essays from the medical school. The undergraduate essays are used primarily to see how well you write and to give the admissions committee some further insight into who you are. The medical school admissions committee is looking at your essays for this same information. But the people reviewing medical school essays are looking at much more. Depending on the particular question, the medical essays tend to fall into one of the following four categories.

- Motivation
- Commitment
- Diligence
- Maturity

Motivation

The first type of medical school question is one that looks at your motivation for becoming a doctor. Are you interested in the healing art of medicine, or is your focus on becoming rich and successful? Hint: the right answer is not "becoming rich and successful." While this may seem obvious, I often see students talk about the prestige of becoming a doctor. Yes, being a doctor can be prestigious. But if that is your focus, then the EAMPs are not going to be impressed.

So, how do you show what your motivation is? Discuss something that has occurred in your life that provides a personal touch. Maybe you were injured as a child and were inspired by the care provided by your doctors. Maybe you watched a relative suffer a debilitating illness and you were impressed by the compassion of the doctors who treated your relative.

You may also show your motivation through the activities in which you have been involved. Are you founder of a group that provides regular visits to nursing home residents? Have you been involved in an activity for several years where the only compensation is the good feeling you receive? These are the sorts of experiences that medical schools are looking for in strong applicants to early admissions programs. Depth of involvement in a particular activity is much more important here than the number of activities that you may have been involved in.

Commitment

The second type of medical essay tries to confirm that you are serious about becoming a doctor and will continue through the early acceptance program if you are accepted. Many students start college planning to go to medical school but never finish the necessarily coursework. This occurs for many reasons including the inability of the student to handle the work but also a lack of motivation when the hard work needs to be done. Medical schools do not want to waste an acceptance on a student who may not be serious about becoming a doctor. In fact, the basic academic requirements to even apply to early acceptance programs are designed to weed out those students who may not be able to handle the academic rigors of the coursework.

Your answers to the essay questions are another way for the medical admissions committee to get a feel for how serious you are about becoming a doctor. There are a number of ways to show the depth of your commitment to becoming a doctor. Most of these we have already discussed, such as doctor shadowing, engaging in scientific research, and volunteering at facilities like clinics and nursing homes. These activities may have been mentioned in the application, but the medical essays often give you the opportunity to expand on your involvement with such activities.

Diligence

A third medical essay topic is one that asks for your interest in the particular program that you are applying to. Medical schools are like colleges in that they want to make sure that you have done your research and are applying to the best programs for your needs. Different medical schools have different focuses, and the burden is on you to convince the medical admissions committee that you are not just applying to every program you can find but rather are applying only to the most appropriate early admissions programs. Each medical school may also have a different focus on how teaching is done. You should match your learning style with a particular medical school.

Examine the different early acceptance programs to see which might be the most appropriate for your interests. Not all programs have a particular focus, but if you are considering an application to one that does have a focus, you want to make sure that your essay reflects your interest in that area.

Maturity

The fourth category of general medical essay is a question that tries to gauge your level of maturity. Medical schools recognize that it takes a high level of maturity to be successful in medical school. It requires even more maturity for students who wish to be successful in an EAMP. To show maturity in your essays, keep the focus on your beliefs and your actions, not on you. Communicate your answer to the question posed by being factual in discussing what you have done.

Now that you know the general topics of medical essays, let's look at some of the actual questions used by early admissions medical programs, either currently or in the past. Northwestern University's Honors Program in Medical Education (HPME) in the past asked three questions on their application.

1. *Explain the factors that are driving you toward a career in medicine.*

    This first question is the classic "why medicine" essay that virtually all of the early acceptance programs ask. While this is probably the most important essay question for you to answer, you can use the same essay at most of the programs.

2. *If you were not attending a school next year and had the freedom to dedicate the year to anything you wanted to do, what would it be?*

    Northwestern's purpose for this question is to both measure your level of maturity and to see what kind of person you are at heart. As with all of these questions, there are no right or wrong answers. What is important is to read each question carefully and answer the question asked. Your answer to a question like this does not need to be that you would spend the year doing scientific research. Tell them what your true passion is and how that passion drives you. If that passion is research, fine. But, if it involves helping those less fortunate, that is fine also.

3. *How did you deal with a situation where you didn't achieve the outcome you desired?*

This is a simple maturity question. There are looking not only for an answer to the question but also for something that you hopefully learned from the experience.

Here is the question from Virginia Commonwealth University.

Comment on your motivation for, and interest in, medicine.
This is the "why medicine" essay. Although the question is phrased differently than Northwestern's first question, they are looking for the same information.

Union College and their program with Albany Medical College ask two questions. The first is as follows:

Albany Medical College seeks uniquely qualified students for the Leadership in Medicine Program. This special program focuses on three key areas that today's physicians must be prepared to address: the economic and financial problems facing medicine, including health policy and health management; the increasing complexity of biomedical ethics; and the need to maintain a global perspective. This intense program prepares physicians to provide excellent health care delivery and to take a leadership role in the rapid transformation occurring in health care management, especially in the areas of medical practice administration, organizational structures, information technology, and comprehensive medical insurance coverage.

The Leadership in Medicine Program educates future physicians not only in the basic and clinical sciences, but also in the business/management/policy side of medicine. Please state why you are applying to this program and what uniquely qualifies you for the special focus of this program.

This question is somewhat unusual in that it doesn't ask for the basic "why medicine" essay. Instead, it focuses on why the student would be a good applicant for their program and the specific focus that this program has. To answer this question you need to examine carefully the focus of the program as described in the preamble to the question. It may also be helpful to examine the web pages associated with the program to see if there is a further explanation of the program's focus.

The second question from the Union–Albany program is:

Describe yourself (other than scholastic achievements). (1000 character limit)

This is a generic question that allows you to enhance your application by focusing on those aspects of your life that make you a strong candidate for an early acceptance program and that have not been previously discussed in your application. Typically this may include some of the volunteer activities you have been involved with although it may also involve a discussion of your personal beliefs.

Siena College also has an EAMP with Albany Medical College. Unlike the program that Union has with Albany Medical College, the Siena College program places emphasis on humanities, ethics, and social service.

Siena's supplemental question reflects this different philosophical approach.

Describe a personal service experience in your high school or community, what you have gained from this experience, and how it reflects the unique values of the Siena College/ Albany Medical College Program.

This question has multiple parts, and you must make sure that you answer all parts of the question. You also need to do your research to make sure you understand what the unique values are of the Siena–Albany program. Typically, you should be able to find information of this type on the colleges' websites.

Here are some examples of questions from other EAMPs. The University of Rochester program has two questions.

1. *Your freshman year in college hasn't started yet, but you're applying for early acceptance to a graduate degree program. Please comment on why you feel you will be ready in a few years for the challenges of your chosen graduate program.* (limit 300)

2. *Please explore the distinct educational philosophy, area of study, or research project of a faculty member teaching in the graduate program to which you are applying. Tell us why you would enjoy working with this person. Rather than contacting a faculty member, please research the variety of print and online resources available.*

Rice University's program has three questions for applicants.

1. *What aspirations, experiences, or relationships have motivated you to study in the eight-year Rice–Baylor Medical Scholars Program?*

2. *Outside of academics, what do you enjoy doing most?*

3. *Describe the most difficult adversity you have faced, and describe how you dealt with it.*

Penn State University has two different questions for applicants.

1. *Write a personal statement indicating why you want to be a physician, why you want an accelerated program and why you've selected this Penn State / Jefferson program.* Please answer this question in 500 words or less.

2. *Describe what you think your strongest qualities are, as well as weaknesses that you would like to improve upon.*

The University of Miami asks one question.

Give a personal history of yourself, your reasons for wanting to study in your chosen field, and why you are interested in the Dual-Degree Honors Program at the University of Miami. (must be 2 pages)

Drexel University asks the following question:

Tell the Admissions Committee why you are applying to the joint program(s) with Drexel University College of Medicine. Be sure to explain why you want to be a physician and more specifically why you want to obtain your medical education at Drexel University College of Medicine. If you are applying to any of our accelerated joint programs (those with only 3 years of college), be sure to explain why you are pursuing that particular option.

The University of Connecticut asks five questions on their application.

1. *Please briefly share the influences on your decision to pursue this field of medicine.*
2. *Please describe your interests, activities, hobbies, etc. outside the area of health sciences.*
3. *Please list your work experiences paid or volunteer while in high school.*
4. *Why are you applying for the combined medical or dental program at the University of Connecticut?*
5. *Fast forward four years. Please describe what you will be like when you are a University of Connecti-*

cut senior. What will have been distinctive about your preparation for professional school?

Brown University's Program in Liberal Medical Education (PLME) asks:

Most high school students are unsure about eventual career choices. What experiences have you to consider medicine as your future profession? Please describe specifically why you have chosen to apply to the Program in Liberal Medical Education in pursuit of your career in medicine. Also, be sure to indicate your rationale on how the PLME is a 'good fit' for your personal academic and future professional goals.

As you can see there is great variation in the questions asked by the different early acceptance programs. Moreover, the medical schools and colleges may change the questions they ask in subsequent years. However, by having some idea of the various types of questions that might be asked, you can start work on general responses before you even decide which programs you are going to apply to. Since your answer to the essay questions can be the difference between an invitation to interview and no interview, taking the additional time to work on essays may make the difference.

Chapter 5

The Medical School Interview

Congratulations! Based on your grades, test scores, activities, and essays, you have been accepted into the undergraduate college you applied to. Upon acceptance, your file is sent to the medical school admissions committee for their review. After the medical school admissions committee has reviewed all of the files, they decide which students to ask for an interview. Only those students who are asked to interview continue to be considered for acceptance into the early acceptance program.

The medical school will contact you directly to arrange a time for an interview. Some medical schools give you several dates to choose from for your interview while other programs give you a specific date for your interview and it is up to you to be there on that date. You should be aware that unlike most college interviews, medical school interviews are always conducted at the campus of the medical college. This means that if you are asked to interview for a particular program, you need to travel to that campus for your interview. It can be expensive to travel to a campus that is far from where you live, particularly if you have multiple interviews. If money is an issue, when deciding where to apply, you should carefully consider if you can afford to attend an interview on a campus far from where you live.

While getting an interview is great news, not all students given an interview will be accepted into a program. In fact, in most programs, far fewer than half of the students interviewed are accepted into the program. In this chapter we are going to look at what you can do to have a great medical school interview and improve your chances of acceptance into an early acceptance program.

Before we discuss what happens during a medical school interview, it is important that you understand what the medical school interviewers look for in a successful candidate. The primary characteristics of a successful candidate are a passion to become a physician, a high level of maturity, and interpersonal skills that allow you to become a compassionate physician. What does that mean?

The interviewers are trying to learn what you are like as a person, how you think, what your values are, and how you handle pressure. What they are evaluating with these interviews is your maturity level. Medical schools want to make sure that you are mature enough to handle the rigors of medical school as well as the rigors of being a practicing physician.

Interviewers are also looking to see how well you communicate with others. The ability to communicate with patients and other doctors is critical to be a successful physician, and your ability to speak is tested directly with the interview. Can you speak clearly and articulately? Can you answer questions in such a way that a patient will understand you?

We will look at some of the specific questions you might be asked during a medical school interview later in this chapter; but first, let's look at the basics of preparing for the medical school interview.

How to Be Successful at a Medical School Interview

There are a number of very basic things that you need to do to make sure that you have a successful medical school interview. Here is a list of things you need to do before even starting your interview:

1. *Confirm where you need to be to begin the interview and get there early.* You do not want to be late to your interview because you didn't know where you were

going. There is no worse way to start an interview than by being late. Plan to arrive at least fifteen minutes before your scheduled interview. Also make sure that you have the proper directions to get to where you are going. Ideally, drive to the interview site the day before the interview to know exactly where you are going.

2. *Prepare for the interview by considering questions you might be asked and your answers to them, as well as questions you wish to have answered.* Later in this chapter I will give you a list of questions that are typically asked in medical school interviews as well as a list of questions that you might consider asking of the people you speak with.

3. *Review your application and in particular all of your activities.* It is common for interviewers to ask a number of detailed questions about your résumé, so you want to make sure that it is fresh in your mind. Be prepared to answer questions about not just what you did, but why you participated in that particular activity and what you learned from your participation.

4. *Learn as much as you can about the medical school you are applying to.* Medical schools, like colleges, may have different teaching styles and different personalities. Is there an emphasis on family practice or is it more of a research based medical facility? What options are there for foreign study during your time in medical school?

5. *Dress appropriately and conservatively.* Suit and tie are always appropriate for men. Women can wear a pants suit or a dress. If you have piercings anywhere other than your ears, right before your interview would be a good time to remove the piercings. If you have tattoos, try to cover them up as much as possible. It is fine to show your individual spirit but piercings and tattoos are not the way to do it for medical school interviews.

6. *Turn off your cell phone before going into the interview.* This is just common courtesy. There should be nothing more important to you at this time than the interview.

7. *Bring multiple copies of your activities résumé with you.* Most interviewers have a copy of your application or activities résumé available to them, but it is always a good idea to bring a copy of your activities résumé in case the interviewer is not fully prepared.

8. *Have a firm handshake when greeting people, but not too firm.* You want to be self-assured, but you don't want to crush their hand.

9. *Look people in the eyes while talking with them.* This is the sign of someone who is self-confident and also indicates that you are interested in what is being said by the person you are interviewing with.

10. *Smile and be positive.* Yes, you are nervous. Yes, these programs are incredibly competitive. But during the interview you need to get past those things and present yourself as the strong candidate that you are. If you were not a strong candidate, you wouldn't even be having the interview.

11. *Listen carefully to the question asked and respond directly to that question.* When people are nervous they don't always listen to the question being asked or they hear the first part of the question and assume they know how the question will end. Don't fall into this trap. By carefully listening to the entire question before formulating your response you will be sure to answer the question that was asked of you.

    If you need a second to collect your thoughts before answering, take a deep breath and answer when you are ready. You should also be aware of how fast you are talking. When someone is nervous it is very common that they talk too fast. Slow it down so that you are having a conversation, not rushing through.

12. *Don't ramble in your answers; keep answers fairly short but responsive.* Giving a long, rambling response to a question generally indicates that you either don't have a succinct logical response or that you are nervous. Preparation is key. Make sure you are adequately prepared to answer most questions you might be asked.

13. *Don't be conceited; be self-assured but humble about your accomplishments.* No one likes someone who comes across as self-centered. At the same time, you should be self–confident and ready to talk about all of the strengths you have and why you would make a good candidate for the program. It can be a fine line to walk between conceited and self-assured. Practice answering questions, with someone who knows you asking typical questions. Ask them to evaluate how you might appear to a stranger.

14. *Make sure that you come across as sincere.* Medical schools are looking for bright, mature students who can handle the work but will also be caring, compassionate physicians. Do not try to fake who you are during the interview. If you try to be someone you are not, the interviewer will most likely pick up on this and will not treat you as a serious candidate.

What Will Happen during a Medical School Interview?

There is no one formula for the medical school interview process, but most interviews follow a standard pattern. You will most likely have a number of interviews during your time on campus. The interviews may just involve you and the interviewer. You may also have several interviewers asking you questions at the same time. Some programs also do group interviews, where a number of prospective applicants are interviewed at the same time.

Most programs arrange for you to interview with a physician who teaches at the medical school. It is also common to interview with students who are currently in the program. The day of your interviews you will be given a tour of the medical school and often a hospital associated with the school. A lunch with students currently in the program is common. Despite the more informal nature of the tour and the lunch, you must keep in mind that the interview process is continuing. Admissions offices commonly ask tour guides or students you had lunch with for their feedback on you as a student in their program. The process of going through multiple interviews and the tour generally takes most of the day, so you should not plan on doing anything other than the interviews on the day they have been arranged.

The Interviewers

I mentioned that you may be interviewed by a physician who teaches in the program or by past or current students of the program. Try to find out before the day of the interview who you will be interviewing with. If you are able to do so, do some research to learn what you can about your interviewer. Where did they go to college and medical school? What is their medical specialty? Have they been involved in research and published papers? Knowing something about your interviewer helps you feel at ease and gives you topics to discuss with your interviewer. It also shows that you are motivated enough to do the research about your interviewer.

Most of the people interviewing you for these combined degree programs will be friendly and trying to put you at ease. They really do want to get to know you to see if you are a good candidate for their program. However, different people use different interviewing techniques. Some questioners may get aggressive during the interview to see how you handle pressure. Don't become upset if this happens to you. Keep your cool, and don't get defensive. Answer the questions in a calm and respectful manner. Medicine can be stressful, and if you are able to remain calm during the interview, it shows that you can handle the stress without breaking down.

Questions You Should Be Prepared to Answer

There are literally thousands of questions that you might be asked during the medical school interview process. But don't panic. Most of the questions fall into a particular category of question. Knowing the major types of questions helps you answer any question you are asked. The first four categories of questions revolve around you and your résumé. Categories five through eight focus more on why you wish to be a doctor. Finally, the interview will end with open-ended questions so you can learn more about the medical school where you are interviewing.

While many interviewers follow this general order in asking questions, there are no rules that they need to follow in asking you questions. Some interviewers jump right into the question of why you wish to become a doctor. Don't worry about the order in which you might be asked questions. Rather, make sure that you understand the categories of questions and that you are prepared to answer questions related to each of the categories, regardless of the order of the questions.

1. General questions about you and your activities

Most questioners will start the interview asking general questions about you and the activities you have participated in during high school. You should carefully review your résumé before attending the interview. Here are typical questions that may be asked about you and your activities:

What do you do for enjoyment?
What are the last three books you read?
What magazines do you read?

What is your greatest strength or weakness?
How do you spend your free time?

2. Questions about your research experiences

Most students who are competitive for BS/MD programs
have some type of research they have participated in before
applying to these programs. You will most likely be asked
questions about the research you did. Typically, you need
to discuss the specifics of what you did during the research,
what the purpose of the research was, and the findings of
the research. The most important point is that you must be
prepared to show you fully understand the nature of your
research project. These questions are meant to confirm that
you have a real interest in the research you engaged in and
did not just do it to enhance your résumé. You may also be
asked to describe a problem you faced when you were con-
ducting the research.

3. Questions about your doctor shadowing experiences

Your application should have detailed your involvement with
following one or more physicians while they were working.
You will most likely be asked questions about this experience including what you did during the shadowing, what
medical problems you were exposed to, and whether the doctors you worked with influenced your outlook on a career in
medicine?
    The types of medical problems you observed are not as
important as the experience you had following the doctor.

4. Questions about your volunteer activities

Most interviewers will ask you questions about your volunteer activities. These questions are important because your
answers tell the interviewer something about your compas-

sion. Compassion is a major factor that BS/MD programs are looking for in applicants. They want students who are concerned about others, and not just about themselves and how much money they can make as a physician. Your answers to these questions allow you to expand on what is hopefully your sincere desire to work for the betterment of others.

You may discuss not only what you did with your volunteer work but also what your motivation was in volunteering at this facility. You might discuss how you felt after volunteering.

Most students have some of their volunteer activities in health-related fields, so you can also use these questions to reinforce your understanding of the health care field and your commitment to becoming a physician.

If you do not have a long-term (more than one year) commitment to a particular volunteer program, and you have a good reason for this, now is your chance to explain why you don't have the long-term involvement.

5. Questions about why you want to be a doctor

Why do you want to be a doctor?

No matter which program you are interviewing for or who is asking the questions, this question, or some variation of it, is the central part of your interview. It is critical that you have a good answer to this question prepared before your interview. Why is this question so important?

This question allows the interviewer to assess your motivation to become a physician. Are you passionate about becoming a physician? Have you really thought about what it means to be a doctor? Do you understand how rigorous the training is and what an effect being a doctor has on your lifestyle? Are you ready, as a high school senior, to commit yourself to a career in medicine?

A similar question that often is asked during an interview is, When did you first decide on medicine as a profession?

Most students applying to BS/MD programs have wanted to become a doctor for many years. What is important in answering this question is that you communicate that you have given a great deal of thought to your chosen profession.

What will you do if you are not admitted to the BS/MD program is another common question that may be asked of you. The best answer is that you will continue to work toward your goal of becoming a doctor by taking the traditional route to medical school. You want to communicate that your ultimate goal is to become a doctor. While you would prefer the BS/MD route, you are not willing to give up your dream just because you might not get into one of these programs.

A related question is, What would you do if you are not accepted into medical school at all? In asking this question, the interviewer is seeing whether you are focused on science-related fields even if medical school is not possible. Your answer does not necessarily need to be employment in a science-related field if your focus is on other fields where you may be able to help people. Remember, passion and compassion.

Here are some other questions that you might be asked that relate to the category of your interest in medicine:

What type of doctor do you want to be and why?
Are you more interested in a clinical practice or research? Why do you have an interest in that type of medicine?
What strengths or qualities do you have that will help make you a good physician?
What qualities should a good physician have?
What do you think you will like about medicine? What will you dislike?
What challenges do you think you will face during your medical career?

You want to establish your passion and compassion. But, it is not enough to use these buzz words. Use stories and examples from your life to show that you have the passion and compassion that will make you a great physician. You do not need to ever even say the words passion and compassion if the stories you tell establish that this is who you are. Think about who you are and how your life exhibits these two traits before the interview. Then let your story do the convincing.

6. Questions about why you want to do a combined BS/MD program rather than the traditional route.

I have already discussed how competitive these programs are and how much of the admissions process revolves around your proving your serious interest in a career in medicine. However, the vast majority of students, including those who have had a dream for years of becoming a doctor, still go the traditional route to become a doctor. Why do you think a combined BS/MD program is preferable for you?

There are many reasons you may think such a program is in your best interest. You may like the accelerated program because it allows you to reach your goal of becoming a physician sooner. Keep in mind, most of these BS/MD programs are not accelerated, and it takes you the traditional eight years to complete college and medical school. If you are applying to an accelerated program, then this answer is fine, but if you are applying to one of the eight-year programs, this type of answer shows that you don't know enough about the program you have applied to.

The most common answer to this type of question is that an early acceptance into medical school takes much of the pressure off you during your college years. You don't have to worry about grades as much as the traditional students, who are competing with each other to see who can get the best grades. As previously mentioned, the minimum grade point averages required of most programs is around a 3.5 GPA. Students who are qualified for these programs rarely have a problem receiving an average 3.5 GPA.

In a BS/MD program, you also have more flexibility to take classes that are of interest to you and that are not just focused on the sciences. Most of the BS/MD programs have no problem with their students taking classes outside the sciences, and in fact many encourage academic exploration. They understand that a well-rounded student will often have an easier time communicating with patients than one who spent all four years of college in a science lab.

Students in these programs often have additional benefits such as early experiences at the medical school or enhanced research experiences. Brown University's Program in Liberal Medical Education (PLME), for instance, has the Medicine in Action program, where undergraduates and medical students can "explore a variety of clinical settings, observe physician/patient relationships firsthand, go on rounds with the medical team, and get to know individual medical school faculty and alumni more closely. Medical students are offered the opportunity to hone their career choices by seeking mentors in their area of interest." Opportunities like this can greatly enhance a student's medical education.

Finally, some programs do not require their students to take the MCAT before medical school, or the required score on the MCAT is eased for those in the program. This alleviates much of the stress related to taking this high stakes test that those not in the program will need to experience.

7. Questions about why you are interested in this particular program

In Chapter 3, I discussed the different types of programs and the unique nature of each program. The questions in this category ensure you have applied to the right program for you. There can be overlap between the answers to these types of questions and those that ask why you want a BS/MD program. For instance, as we just discussed, the PLME program at Brown provides certain additional program options for its students. You should investigate what additional educational opportunities each program makes available so that you are prepared to discuss your interest in that type of program.

Some BS/MD programs also have a particular focus, and if you have an interest in the focus of that program, now is the time to discuss your interest. For instance, Union College and Albany Medical College have a joint BS/MD program known as the Leadership in Medicine Program. This program emphasizes undergraduate training in the sciences as well as humanities and health care management. This would be a good program for those students interested in medicine as well as health care management.

Albany Medical College also has a program with Rensselaer Polytechnic Institute called the Physician Scientist Program. This seven-year program has a goal to "prepare physicians who will advance the practice of medicine through their clinical skills combined with their understanding and ability to carry out health care research."

Although each of these programs uses Albany Medical College, it should be clear that a single student would not likely be a good choice for both programs. Choosing the right programs to apply to becomes particularly important when this question is asked of you. And if you think you can just fake an answer, the interviewer is looking at your entire résumé to see if it is consistent with the focus of this program. If you claim to have an interest in the Rensselaer program, your résumé should contain several examples of your interest in scientific research.

Here are some examples of questions that you might be asked, to determine whether this is the right program for you.

Why are you applying to this BS/MD program and in particular this medical school?
Where else have you applied?

What's your first choice and why?

What qualities do you have that other applicants don't?

How are you a good match for our medical school?

What makes you unique?

What criteria are you using to evaluate potential medical schools?

8. Questions about current medical issues and ethics

Most interviewers will ask you at least one question related to a current topic in medical ethics. Common topics include embryonic stem cell research, medical malpractice, socialized medicine, genetic engineering, abortion, physician assisted suicide, euthanasia and other end of life issues.

There are several purposes for these questions. First, the interviewer is seeing whether you have knowledge of current medical issues. Most students who have a passion for medicine will have given at least some thought to issues related to controversial topics.

Second, the interviewer is looking to see if you have the ability to think logically about different topics. Note that these types of questions are not focused on what your opinion might be on the topic. Most ethical questions do not have right or wrong answers. But you do need to have some sort of opinion and have a logical basis for your opinion.

Third, your cultural sensitivity and bias are being examined. Do you have the maturity to understand that people with different cultural or spiritual backgrounds may view these topics very differently? Do you understand that even if you do not agree with someone's belief, that it is their right to have that belief?

Related questions might include the following:

What's the biggest issue facing medicine today?

How far do you believe a doctor's responsibility extends to his or her patients?

What changes would you like to see made in the current
  health care system?

Do you think that HIV education in the U.S. and Africa
  can make a difference?

9. Other questions

Some interviewers ask questions that don't seem to have any
relevance to your application. If you are asked one of these
off the wall questions, just relax and give the best answer
you can. The key is to not get flustered. Interviewers are
looking to see how you react to a difficult question, and how
you reason your way through a problem. Again, the issue
here is not whether you give the right answer. You will do
fine as long as you maintain your composure and answer as
best as you can.

10. Final questions

Most interviews will end with the simple question, "Do you
have any questions?" You should always be prepared to ask
at least several questions of the interviewer. These should
be questions that cannot otherwise be answered by looking
at the medical school's website. The only time you might not
need to ask questions at this time is if you have been asking questions as the interview has progressed. If you have
been asking questions of your interviewer and have received
all of the answers to your questions, then you can tell the
interviewer that they have already answered all of your
questions.

Some interviewers will ask if you want to add anything.
If you are asked this question, you should be prepared to
give a short, closing statement emphasizing why you would
be a good candidate for that program. In summarizing
your case, keep in mind ways to reinforce your passion and
compassion.

Here are some possible questions to help you think about what you may wish to ask:

What student support services are available?

What research opportunities might you have?

How are students evaluated during their clinical rotations?

Are there particular strengths in the hospitals associated with the medical school?

How successful is the medical school in placing students into one of their top residency matches?

What is the breakdown of specialties of students who finish the program?

If the medical school does not require BS/MD students to take the MCAT, does the interviewer still recommend you take the MCAT?

What are typical scores that students in the program receive if they take the MCAT?

Final Thoughts

Preparation is the key to a successful interview. If you have seriously read through this chapter, have understood the categories of questions you might be asked, and have thought about answers to each of the categories, you should be well prepared for your interview. During the interview keep two key words in the back of your head; passion and compassion. In answering each question consider how your answer demonstrates your passion for becoming a physician and the compassion that will make you a great physician.

And don't forget to thank the interviewer.

Chapter 6

Paying for Early Medical Programs

Four years of college followed by four years of medical school is very expensive. Even if you are looking at one of the programs that is six or seven years long, there is a tremendous cost associated with medical school. If you are fortunate to come from a family that can easily afford this, then skip ahead to Chapter 7. Otherwise, let's talk about paying for college and medical school.

Paying for College

There are three types of financial aid for college: grants or scholarships, loans, and work-study.

GRANTS AND SCHOLARSHIPS are free money that you do not need to pay back. Most grants and scholarships come from the federal and state government or from the individual college.

LOANS need to be paid back after college. There are many loan programs available from the federal and state governments. Most of these loans have fairly low interest rates. There are also private loans available, although these generally have a higher interest rate and are much less desirable.

WORK-STUDY is a job offered on the campus of the college.

You also need to understand the difference between need-based aid and merit-based aid.

NEED-BASED AID is given by all colleges to students who have need. Anyone who can't pay the full cost of the college has need. A form called the Free Application for Federal Student Aid (FAFSA) determines the amount of need for federal grants and scholarships. Many highly selective colleges also require a form known as the CSS Profile form. The FAFSA form is filled out after January 1 of the year you will first attend college.

The FAFSA and Profile forms ask questions about your and your parents' income, using information that you gave on your tax returns. These forms also ask questions about the amount of money you have in savings or investments. The Profile form is more detailed than the FAFSA form. The government uses the FAFSA form to determine how much your family can pay for college. This is your expected family contribution or your EFC. Your EFC is the same regardless of the cost of the college. Similarly, the individual colleges who use the Profile use that form to determine what your family can pay for college.

Your need is the cost of the college you are looking at minus your EFC. For example, if you are looking at a college that costs $20,000 a year and your EFC is $5,000, your need at that college is $15,000. If you are looking at a college that costs $50,000 a year your EFC is still $5,000, your need at this college is $45,000.

MERIT-BASED AID includes scholarships typically for students who have good grades or have some other special talent such as athletic or musical talent. Most highly selective colleges offer little or no merit-based aid.

Finally, in looking at colleges you should ignore the cost of the college. Yes, you read that right. Ignore the stated cost of the college when you are first deciding which colleges to investigate further. You will see why later in this chapter.

So now you know the basics. However, each college handles financial aid a bit differently. You need to understand how the particular colleges you are looking at handle financial aid. To know that, you need to ask some questions.

Question 1: What percent of my need do you meet?

Remember that EFC, or expected family contribution that the FAFSA determined? Some colleges will meet one hundred percent of your need. Need again is defined as the cost of the college minus your EFC. So what does it mean if a college says they will meet one hundred percent of your need? It means that once the FAFSA or Profile form has determined how much you can pay for college, the college will pay the rest of the bill.

Colleges typically meet the need you have using a combination of grants, loans, and work-study. Most colleges award work-study and loans first, and if there is a need after that, the remaining need is supplied by grants. The colleges typically have a standard loan and work-study amount that they award, and you should ask about what these numbers are when investigating the college.

Let's see an example of a financial aid award from a college that provides one hundred percent of need, with a student who has an EFC of $5,000.

Total cost of college	$50,000
Family's expected contribution	5,000
Need	45,000
Financial aid award	
Work-study	2,000
Loans	4,000
Grants	39,000

At a college that meets one hundred percent of your need you pay $5,000.

But what happens if the college doesn't meet 100% of need?

Many less selective colleges don't pay the total amount of need that their students have under their need-based aid programs. Keep in mind that when I talk about a less selective college, I am talking about a regular application to a college, not one for a college's BS/MD program. Many undergraduate colleges that have BS/MD programs are not very selective for their regular admissions. In most colleges, financial aid is handled the same for its regular applicants and those applying to the BS/MD program.

Let's use the example of our imaginary college from above, only this time assume that the school only provides eighty percent of need.

Total cost of college	$50,000
Family's expected contribution	5,000
Need	45,000

This college only provides eighty percent of the $45,000 need or $36,000. Thus, your out-of-pocket expenses are the $5,000 EFC plus an additional $9,000, for a total cost of $14,000.

This example makes it easy to see why a school that meets one hundred percent of need is often a better financial aid deal than a school that doesn't meet all of the family's need.

Many of the most expensive private colleges meet one hundred percent of the student's need, while cheaper public colleges usually meet less than one hundred percent of the need. This means that for many students it can be cheaper to go to an expensive private college than to attend a cheaper state school. Until you know what percent of need the college meets, don't eliminate a college from consideration just because it is expensive.

Question 2: Do you have merit-based aid?

Many colleges that don't meet one hundred percent of a student's need do offer scholarships for some students. If you are near the top of the application pool for a less selective college, you may get some money if you qualify for merit-based aid. At most colleges that offer a BS/MD program, the applicants to these programs are among the most talented students at that college, and they will often be considered for merit-based aid. Here are some questions you should ask if the college provides merit aid.

How many merit awards are available?

What is the value of the merit awards available?

What are the qualifications to receive one of these merit awards?

This works even for families that don't qualify for need-based aid at all. If you can qualify for a merit-based award, you won't need to pay the full stated cost of the college.

Question 3: How is financial aid determined after the first year?

Some colleges have a policy of providing good financial aid for the first year and then substantially reducing the grant aid in the following years while increasing the loans. You should ask the college in which you are interested how they determine financial aid after the first year and what the average loan is after the first year. While it is typical that the amount of loans will increase each year, if the increase is substantial, you want to take that into consideration.

Question 4: What is the average loan amount at graduation of those students who have loans?

This question will give you the best indication of the amount of loans that this college requires compared to other colleges in which you may be interested. Although most students will have some loans when they graduate, you don't want this amount to be any more than necessary. This is particularly true for students who plan to go to medical school, as loans are the primary form of financial aid for medical school.

Question 5: What is your policy regarding outside scholarships?

Most colleges subtract money earned in outside scholarships from your financial aid package. Some colleges reduce the loan burden by the amount of the scholarship, but other colleges reduce your grant money. If the college reduces the amount of loans you have to take out, that is a benefit to you. There is no benefit to you if the college reduces the grant aid.

Question 6: What is your packaging policy?

Most colleges give a financial aid package that includes grant money, loans, and work-study. But each college combines this money differently. Specifically you want to know:

What percentage of an aid package from your college is grant vs. self-help (that is, loans and work-study)?

The greater amount of grants relative to loans and work-study, the better for the student.

Paying for Medical School

At most medical schools, the primary way of paying for your education is through loans. Most loans are available from the federal government, although many states also have loans available. To qualify for these loans, you need to complete the FAFSA. In calculating your qualification for loans, most colleges do not expect any contribution from your family.

At some of the most selective schools, there are grants available to help pay for medical school. Such grants are available to those families with lower income levels. However, medical schools that have grant money available generally consider the income and assets of the student's parents and not just the student.

At a few of the medical schools that have grant money available, families with lower income levels may not have to contribute as much to the education as would otherwise be the case. For example, Harvard Medical School expects no family contribution from parents with income less than $120,000. However, this sort of financial aid is the exception when dealing with paying for medical school.

The majority of students paying for medical school will do so using loans entirely. Although this may seem like a huge burden, and it is, the expectation is that once medical students graduate and start making money, they will have enough resources to pay off the loans.

Chapter 7

Other Issues
Related to BS/MD Admissions

Acceptance of International Students into Early Acceptance Programs

Many international students are interested in admissions to BS/MD programs, but there are limited options for these students. Most of the BS/MD programs only accept students who are United States citizens or permanent residents of the United States.

There are a few BS/MD programs that consider inter-national students, including the program at Northwestern University and the program at Brown University. International applicants should keep in mind that as competitive as these programs are for U.S. citizens, they are even more competitive for international students. International students who are interested in applying to the few programs available to them must also have other plans for college made, in case they are not accepted into one of the BS/MD programs.

The appendix lists information on each of the BS/MD programs in the U.S., including a note for those that will consider international students.

Acceptance of Transfer Students

Most BS/MD programs only accept applications from students who are incoming freshmen. Transfer applications

73

are specifically not accepted. A limited number of BS/MD programs accept transfer students. Those that do accept transfer students typically do so only after the first year of undergraduate education. Those programs that consider transfer applications are noted in the appendix.

How Many Programs Should You Apply To?

There is no magic number of BS/MD programs that a student should apply to. Contrary to popular belief, more is not necessarily better. While the typical program may only accept one out of twenty students who apply, that does not mean that if you apply to twenty programs you will get into at least one.

Just like choosing a regular college, you want to look at what you want from a college, or BS/MD program, and then find programs that fit your needs. Remember Chapter 3, where I discussed what to look for in a program. That is your starting point. The typical student with whom I work applies to eight to ten BS/MD programs. You should also consider applying to four to six regular colleges that have a strong history of science education and medical school placement. While twelve to fifteen colleges is a huge number of applications, and many more than I recommend for students looking at traditional colleges, it is a good number to consider based on my experiences with students applying to BS/MD programs.

Applying to Traditional College Programs

One final, but very important, note. Because the BS/MD programs are so competitive, every student applying to such a program must also apply to several traditional four-year colleges in case they are not accepted into a BS/MD program. The regular college list should include some colleges in which you are fairly sure you will gain acceptance. These are colleges that many people refer to as safety schools. It should not be a problem to find some good colleges for this purpose, since students who are competitive for BS/MD programs are such strong students.

The focus on the search for traditional colleges should be on colleges that have historically done well in educating their students and preparing them for medical school. This list often includes smaller liberal arts colleges, which are among the most successful colleges in medical school placement.

Some students will want to apply only to the BS/MD programs, with the thought that they are likely to be ad-mitted to most of the undergraduate programs even if they are not admitted to the BS/MD program. They figure that they can always just attend the undergraduate college of the BS/MD program as their college option. This is generally not a good idea. Although some of the undergraduate programs are by themselves good schools to prepare for medical school, many of the undergraduate programs associated with the BS/MD programs are not as academically strong. I strongly advise my students to consider the regular college list as completely separate from the BS/MD list. This way, they are more likely to have regular colleges on their list that do a good job of preparation for medical school rather than colleges that might do an okay job of preparation for medical school.

Programs by State

The information provided in the appendix is believed to be accurate as of the date of the publication of this book. However, BS/MD programs are constantly being started while others are being discontinued. Also, the information regarding minimal grades and test scores as well as the dates applications are required are subject to change at any time. If you find a program in which you have an interest, go to the website of that program to verify information. For updated information you can check my website: www.collegeadmissionspartners.com/bsmd-admissions/.

There is some inconsistency in the way GPA and test scores are reported. Some schools list only their minimum requirements. Some list the averages for *accepted* students. Others list the averages for *enrolled* students. These two averages are not interchangeable. Typically the averages for accepted students are higher than those for enrolled students.

NOTE ON FINANCIAL AID AND COSTS Information about financial aid is listed only if there is a special program available for students admitted to the program. The listed costs are generally for tuition and fees only, although some programs include room and board costs as part of a total package. For more detail about the cost of each program, see the website of each school.

The information provided regarding each school varies in depth depending on the information made available to me by the different programs. Some are more transparent than others and may have more information. I have updated admissions information where available. If current information was not available, I left the information from 2010–2011 academic year.

NOTE ON THE ARRANGEMENT OF THIS APPENDIX Programs are alphabetical by the state where the medical school is, and then alphabetical by associated undergraduate college.

COLLEGE
University of Alabama

MEDICAL SCHOOL
University of Alabama School of Medicine

ADDRESS
UAB Honors Academy, HUC 531
University of Alabama at Birmingham
1530 Third Avenue South
Birmingham, Alabama 35294-1150
205-996-9842
http://main.uab.edu/show.asp?durki=27435

NAME OF PROGRAM
Early Medical School Acceptance Program

LENGTH OF PROGRAM
8 years

APPLICATION DEADLINE
You must be admitted to the university and complete the honors application by December 15. Note: to be considered for scholarship money, you must be admitted by December 1.

INFORMATION ABOUT THE PROGRAM
This program is one of the best values for the undergraduate portion of the program. The program offers in-state students scholarships that pay for the undergraduate tuition; out-of-state students also receive generous scholarships.

The program has a medical school professor teaching freshman seminars to students in the program. This professor also works with students to help them through the entire eight-year program.

Students may major in any of the fifty-three majors offered by the college. Regardless of your major, the program will also make sure you fulfill the prerequisites for the medical school.

Special seminars are offered to students in the program, and a student is required to take at least two seminars before medical school. The seminars focus on themes such as medical ethics, reproductive biology, and the history of medicine. Quarterly meetings provide an opportunity to discuss health care issues and to talk with alumni of the program.

Numerous clinical experiences are made available, including research, patient care, doctor shadowing, and work in laboratories. Students in the program may also receive a summer scholarship to work at local medical facilities. Volunteer service at a local health care facility is required as part of the program.

There is some attrition with this program. About fifteen percent of the students admitted to the program fail out. In addition, about fifty percent are on probation at some time during the undergraduate years.

TRANSFER STUDENTS CONSIDERED

No

CITIZENSHIP REQUIREMENTS

U.S. citizen or permanent resident visa

MINIMUM REQUIRED FACTORS IN SELECTION

CLASSES

Four years of English and math, one year of chemistry or physics, and one year of biology

GPA

3.5 unweighted

SAT

1,340 critical reading and math

ACT

30

2011–2012 ACCEPTANCES

	In State	Out of State	Total
Applicants			
Interviewed			28
New students	5	3	8

FACTORS REQUIRED TO CONTINUE IN PROGRAM

3.5 or higher GPA in natural science and math courses; overall GPA of 3.6 or higher

MCAT REQUIRED

Yes; minimum score of 28

FINANCIAL AID

No special financial aid for students in the program

COST

	Resident Tuition and Fees ($)	Non Resident Tuition and Fees ($)
Undergraduate	8,400	19,230
Medical school	23,321	59,783

COLLEGE

University of South Alabama

MEDICAL SCHOOL

University of South Alabama College of Medicine

ADDRESS

University of South Alabama
Meisler Hall, Room 2500
Mobile, Alabama 36688-0022
251-460-6141
www.southalabama.edu/admissions/honors.html

NAME OF PROGRAM

College of Medicine Early Acceptance Program

LENGTH OF PROGRAM

8 years

APPLICATION DEADLINE

December 15. All materials for application must be received by
this date.

INFORMATION ABOUT THE PROGRAM

After the application deadline the program will select 40 to 45
students for consideration all of whom will be required to attend
an interview at the University of South Alabama. Letters of recommendation are not considered by this program.

Students in the program are required to participate for four
semesters in a course entitled Career Planning: Clinical Observa-
tion. Students are given the opportunity to participate in a two-
week summer clerkship in a clinical setting. The purpose of the
clerkship is to provide a positive clinical experience with a practicing physician.

Students in the program will be reviewed at the end of each
year by the Health Pre-Professions Advisor and a committee of
admissions from the medical school to confirm that academic requirements have been met.

TRANSFER STUDENTS CONSIDERED

No

CITIZENSHIP REQUIREMENTS

U.S. citizen or permanent resident visa. Preference is given to residents of Alabama and certain areas of Florida and Mississippi.
Non-Alabama residents must establish Alabama residency while
in the undergraduate program.

MINIMUM REQUIRED FACTORS IN SELECTION

CLASSES

No specific requirement

GPA

3.5 unweighted

SAT

1,250 critical reading and math

ACT

28

2010–2011 ACCEPTANCES

	In State	Out of State	Total
Applicants	78	50	128
Interviewed	31	14	45
New students	11	4	15

FACTORS REQUIRED TO CONTINUE IN PROGRAM

3.4 or higher GPA in natural science and math courses; overall GPA of 3.5 or higher

MCAT REQUIRED

Yes; minimum score of 29

FINANCIAL AID

There are special financial aid funds for students in the program

COST

	Resident Tuition and Fees ($)	Non Resident Tuition and Fees ($)
Undergraduate	7,950	15,900
Medical school	24,077	47,727

COLLEGE
Caltech

MEDICAL SCHOOL
University of California San Diego School of Medicine

ADDRESS
Caltech Undergraduate Admissions
383 S. Hill Avenue
MC 10-90
Pasadena, California 91125-3405
626-395-6341
http://admissions.caltech.edu/documents
/93-medscholarswithimages2012.pdf

NAME OF PROGRAM
Medical Scholars Program

LENGTH OF PROGRAM
8 years

APPLICATION DEADLINE
November 1. Students must not apply to other single-choice early-action programs.

INFORMATION ABOUT THE PROGRAM
Students in the program will have the opportunity to attend special lectures on medical topics. Summer research activities are also offered with UC San Diego School of Medicine faculty.

TRANSFER STUDENTS CONSIDERED
No

CITIZENSHIP REQUIREMENTS
International students are considered.

MINIMUM REQUIRED FACTORS IN SELECTION

None listed

2010–2011 ACCEPTANCES

	In State	Out of State	Total
Applicants			
Interviewed			
New students			6

No other information provided

FACTORS REQUIRED TO CONTINUE IN PROGRAM

3.5 GPA

MCAT REQUIRED

No

FINANCIAL AID

No special financial aid for students in the program. It should be noted, however, that Caltech generally has strong need-based financial aid.

COST

	Resident Tuition and Fees ($)	Non Resident Tuition and Fees ($)
Undergraduate	39,588	39,588
Medical school	31,431	43,676

COLLEGE

University of California San Diego

MEDICAL SCHOOL

University of California San Diego School of Medicine

ADDRESS

Director of Medical Scholars Program
University of California, San Diego School of Medicine
Office of Admissions, 0621
9500 Gilman Drive
La Jolla, California 92093-0621
858-534-3880
http://meded.ucsd.edu/index.cfm//asa/admissions
/medical_scholars_program//med_scholars_application_process/

NAME OF PROGRAM

UCSD Medical Scholars Program

LENGTH OF PROGRAM

8 years

APPLICATION DEADLINE

Application must be filed between November 1 and November 30.

INFORMATION ABOUT THE PROGRAM

Application to the program is by invitation only. All students who meet the basic academic requirements will be invited to apply to the program. Students in the program are allowed to choose any major. They are only required to complete basic medical school admission requirements. The program is designed to allow students to explore their own interests including student life programs, volunteer efforts, or undergraduate research. The program is somewhat unusual in that it permits students to apply to other medical schools if they wish.

First year students are assigned a medical school student and faculty member as mentors. They provide advice, encouragement, and research opportunities to the student. The program sponsors the Healing Hearts Across Borders program, offering health checkups, medication, food, and clothing to the poor of Tijuana, Mexico. Students in the program have the opportunity to volunteer at the student-run free clinic, conduct undergraduate research at the school of medicine, and get clinical experience through doctor shadowing.

TRANSFER STUDENTS CONSIDERED

No

CITIZENSHIP REQUIREMENTS

U.S. citizen or permanent resident visa; California resident

MINIMUM REQUIRED FACTORS IN SELECTION

CLASSES

No specific requirement

GPA

4.0 weighted GPA as calculated on the UC application; average entering student GPA is 4.26

SAT

2,250

ACT

34

2011–2012 ACCEPTANCES

	In State	Out of State	Total
Applicants	500+		500±
Interviewed	25		25
New students	12		12

FACTORS REQUIRED TO CONTINUE IN PROGRAM

Overall GPA of 3.5 or higher and a 3.5 GPA in upper division science and humanities/social sciences; minimum six quarters of humanities or social science courses with an emphasis on literature and composition

MCAT REQUIRED

No

FINANCIAL AID

No special financial aid for students in the program

COST

	Resident Tuition and Fees ($)	Non Resident Tuition and Fees ($)
Undergraduate	13,234	not applicable
Medical school	31,431	not applicable

COLLEGE
University of Colorado Denver

MEDICAL SCHOOL
University of Colorado School of Medicine

ADDRESS
University of Colorado Denver School of Medicine
BA/BS-MD Program
13001 East 17th Place, Room C1009
Mail Stop C297
Aurora, Colorado 80045
303-352-3557
www.ucdenver.edu/academics/colleges/CLAS/BachelorsPrograms
/ProgramsDegrees/BABSMD/Pages/home.aspx

NAME OF PROGRAM
BA/BS-MD Program

LENGTH OF PROGRAM
8 years

APPLICATION DEADLINE
November 12; date varies each year. Undergraduate application
should be submitted by October 5.

INFORMATION ABOUT THE PROGRAM
The program admits students from a diverse background who are
committed to serving the health care needs of Colorado. Students
may major in any subject offered by the university. The summer
before starting college students participate in a one-week bridge
program. In the summer after freshman year students spend
eight weeks working in hospitals or clinics in the Denver area.
The summer after sophomore year students participate in a research practicum. The summer after junior year students participate in an MCAT prep course. Students are paid for their time in
the summer programs.

TRANSFER STUDENTS CONSIDERED
No

CITIZENSHIP REQUIREMENTS
U.S. citizen or permanent resident visa; Colorado residents only

MINIMUM REQUIRED FACTORS IN SELECTION

CLASSES
No specific requirement

GPA
3.5 and a CCHE score of 110 or better

SAT
1,050

ACT
23

2010–2011 ACCEPTANCES

	In State	Out of State	Total
Applicants			
Interviewed			
New students	8 to 10		8 to 10

No other information provided

FACTORS REQUIRED TO CONTINUE IN PROGRAM
3.5 overall GPA with no grade lower than B in any medical school prerequisite course

MCAT REQUIRED
Yes; minimum score of 28

FINANCIAL AID
No special financial aid for students in the program, although special help is provided by the financial aid office to find additional aid

COST

	Resident Tuition and Fees ($)	Non Resident Tuition and Fees ($)
Undergraduate	4,318	not applicable
Medical school	32,683	not applicable

COLLEGE
University of Connecticut at Storrs

MEDICAL SCHOOL
University of Connecticut School of Medicine

ADDRESS
Special Programs in Medicine and Dental Medicine
University of Connecticut
2131 Hillside Road, U-88
Storrs, Connecticut 06269-3088
860-486-3137
http://medicine.uchc.edu/prospective/babs_md/

NAME OF PROGRAM
B.A./B.S. and M.D. Combined Program in Medicine

LENGTH OF PROGRAM
8 years

APPLICATION DEADLINE
December 1 for college. Program supplemental application due
January 1.

INFORMATION ABOUT THE PROGRAM
Students are allowed to complete any major offered by the university, and students are encouraged to explore a wide range of undergraduate courses. As undergraduates, students in the program
are offered opportunities to engage in research and clinical experiences. This may include summer research at the UConn health
center, clinical experience at the school of medicine, attendance at
research meetings, and community service activities through the
health center.

TRANSFER STUDENTS CONSIDERED
No

CITIZENSHIP REQUIREMENTS
International students considered. Connecticut students given
preference in admissions.

MINIMUM REQUIRED FACTORS IN SELECTION

CLASSES

No specific requirement

GPA

3.5 unweighted

SAT

1,300, 650 minimum on critical reading and 650 minimum on math

ACT

29

2010–2011 ACCEPTANCES

	In State	Out of State	Total
Applicants	93	139	232
Interviewed	26	16	42
New students	12	3	15

FACTORS REQUIRED TO CONTINUE IN PROGRAM

3.6 GPA; participation in clinical, research, and community activities; and a favorable interview with the medical school during the senior year of college

MCAT REQUIRED

Yes; minimum score of 30 with section scores of 8 or better

FINANCIAL AID

All enrolled students considered for merit-based scholarships.

COST

	Resident Tuition and Fees ($)	Non Resident Tuition and Fees ($)
Undergraduate	11,362	29,124
Medical school	30,879	57,051

COLLEGE

George Washington University

MEDICAL SCHOOL

George Washington University School of Medicine
and Health Sciences

ADDRESS

Office of Undergraduate Admissions
The George Washington University
2121 I Street NW Suite 201
Washington, DC 20052
202-994-6040
http://undergraduate.admissions.gwu.edu/seven-year-bamd

NAME OF PROGRAM

Seven Year BA/MD Program

LENGTH OF PROGRAM

7 years

APPLICATION DEADLINE

December 1

INFORMATION ABOUT THE PROGRAM

To apply for the program a student must submit the Honors, Accelerated and Special Programs application of the Common Application Supplement.

Freshmen are encouraged to live together in the same dormitory. Seminars and health care experiences are made available to students in the program. Students may arrange their program to have a period of study abroad. During the first three years of the program, a student must complete a major and meet all general curriculum requirements. A community service project is required each year. Students are supported by an undergraduate BA/MD advisor, the assistant dean of admissions at the school of medicine, and student mentors in the program. Progress through the program is reviewed annually. This program is unusual, as the BA degree is awarded at the end of the three-year undergraduate experience.

A review committee meets at the end of the third year to make a final recommendation regarding admission to the medical school. This recommendation will be given if the student has met all of the requirements of the program.

TRANSFER STUDENTS CONSIDERED

No

CITIZENSHIP REQUIREMENTS

U.S. citizen or permanent resident visa; Canadian citizens also considered

MINIMUM REQUIRED FACTORS IN SELECTION

CLASSES

No specific requirement

GPA

No specific requirement; competitive students will be in the top ten percent of their high school class.

SAT

No specific requirement; competitive scores are 2,100 and higher; SAT subject exam in one of the sciences and one in math

ACT

No specific requirement

2010–2011 ACCEPTANCES

	In State	Out of State	Total
Applicants		700	700
Interviewed		50	50
New students		10	10

FACTORS REQUIRED TO CONTINUE IN PROGRAM

Overall 3.6 GPA; minimum grade of B in courses required for admission to medical school; completion of a major at the college

MCAT REQUIRED

No

FINANCIAL AID

Students in the program pay a special fixed tuition rate with an annual merit discount for the first three years of the program.

COST

	Resident Tuition and Fees ($)	Non Resident Tuition and Fees ($)
Undergraduate	45,780	45,780
Medical school	51,278	51,278

COLLEGE

St. Bonaventure

MEDICAL SCHOOL

George Washington University School of Medicine and Health Sciences

ADDRESS

Director, Franciscan Health Care Professions
Biology Department, De La Roche Hall Room 219
St. Bonaventure, New York 14778
716-375-2656; email preferred to aknowles@sbu.edu
www.sbu.edu/about_sbu.aspx?id=6230

NAME OF PROGRAM

Dual Admission BS/MD 4+4

LENGTH OF PROGRAM

8 years

APPLICATION DEADLINE

Dec. 1; the basic application should be completed by November 1.

INFORMATION ABOUT THE PROGRAM

Qualified applicants are invited for an interview at St. Bonaventure in January. Students who pass this interview are invited for an interview at the George Washington Medical School in late February to early March. Acceptance decisions are made in mid to late March.

Community service is taken into consideration for admission to the program. At least two teacher recommendations are required, and one of them must be from a science teacher. Letters from non-teachers, such as employers, coaches, or volunteer coordinators, are encouraged. These letters should briefly discuss the writer's personal knowledge of and experience with the student.

You are required to write one or two personal statements outlining your interest in medicine and your particular interest in St. Bonaventure and George Washington University.

A résumé of all of your extracurricular activities is also required.

TRANSFER STUDENTS CONSIDERED

No

CITIZENSHIP REQUIREMENTS

U.S. citizen or permanent resident visa; Canadian citizens also considered

MINIMUM REQUIRED FACTORS IN SELECTION

CLASSES

No specific requirement

GPA

90 or higher

SAT

1,300 critical reading and math; SAT subject exam in biology (M is preferred); chemistry is acceptable

ACT

29

2011–2012 ACCEPTANCES

	In State	Out of State	Total
Applicants			170
Interviewed			63
New students			10

FACTORS REQUIRED TO CONTINUE IN PROGRAM

Must be a full-time student; minimum 3.6 GPA in all science courses and overall; grade of B– or better in all courses; completion of core science and English requirements; maintaining character and comportment requirements

MCAT REQUIRED

No

FINANCIAL AID

Scholarship is available for the undergraduate years.

COST

	Resident Tuition and Fees ($)	Non Resident Tuition and Fees ($)
Undergraduate	28,727	28,727
Medical school	50,903	50,903

COLLEGE
Howard University

MEDICAL SCHOOL
Howard University College of Medicine

ADDRESS
Preprofessional Advisor
Center for Preprofessional Education
College of Arts and Sciences
2225 Georgia Avenue NW Room 518
Howard University
Washington, DC 20059-1014
202-238-2363
www.coas.howard.edu/preprofessionaleducation

NAME OF PROGRAM
Howard University College of Medicine Joint Degree Program

LENGTH OF PROGRAM
6 years

APPLICATION DEADLINE
March 1

INFORMATION ABOUT THE PROGRAM
This is a modified BS/MD program that accepts students during the senior year of high school or the freshman year of college. Besides academics, the admissions committee considers superior writing skills, maturity, positive self-confidence, leadership skills, and volunteer efforts.

While students may be admitted to the program as high school seniors, they are reevaluated for admission to the medical program after taking the MCAT in April of the sophomore year. At that time the committee also considers whether the student has shown a high level of maturity and a strong commitment to working in an area where there is a shortage of physicians.

TRANSFER STUDENTS CONSIDERED
No

CITIZENSHIP REQUIREMENTS
U.S. citizen or permanent resident visa

MINIMUM REQUIRED FACTORS IN SELECTION

CLASSES

Two years of a foreign language, biology, chemistry, physics, algebra, geometry, and trigonometry.

GPA

3.5 minimum and top five percent of high school class; average 3.7 GPA for students accepted into program

SAT

1,950; average of 2,250 for students accepted into program

ACT

26; average above 30

2010–2011 ACCEPTANCES

	In State	Out of State	Total
Applicants	22	73	95
Interviewed	8	20	28
New students	2	10	12

FACTORS REQUIRED TO CONTINUE IN PROGRAM

Minimum science GPA 3.25, overall GPA 3.50, MCAT score 24

MCAT REQUIRED

Yes, minimum 24

FINANCIAL AID

No special financial aid for students in the program

COST

	Resident Tuition and Fees ($)	Non Resident Tuition and Fees ($)
Undergraduate	21,450	21,450
Medical school	41,215	41,215

COLLEGE

Florida Atlantic University

MEDICAL SCHOOL

Charles E. Schmidt College of Medicine

ADDRESS

Harriet L. Wilkes Honors College
Florida Atlantic University
Office of Admissions
5353 Parkside Drive
Jupiter, Florida 33458-2906
561-799-8646
www.fau.edu/divdept/honcol/admissions_med.htm

NAME OF PROGRAM

Wilkes Medical Scholars Program

LENGTH OF PROGRAM

7 years

APPLICATION DEADLINE

February 1

INFORMATION ABOUT THE PROGRAM

Three applications are required for this program. Students must apply to the university, the Honors College, and the College of Medicine, the application for which includes two short essays. Students must be accepted into the honors program to be considered for the medical program. Students may major in many different areas within the liberal arts and sciences. Students may, with permission of the program, take four years for the undergraduate portion of the program to broaden their educational experiences.

Part of the curriculum includes medical electives and experiential programs during the year to prepare them for medical school. Students are expected to participate in patient care experiences each summer of their undergraduate years. Students who apply to other medical schools will lose their guaranteed spot at the medical school but may apply as regular applicants. This is a new program that just began in 2011.

The program recommends that applicants have experience with patient interaction.

TRANSFER STUDENTS CONSIDERED

No

CITIZENSHIP REQUIREMENTS

U.S. citizen or permanent resident visa. Student must be a resident of Florida.

MINIMUM REQUIRED FACTORS IN SELECTION

CLASSES

Four years of English and math and one year each of biology and chemistry at a high school in the U.S.

GPA

3.75 unweighted

SAT

1,350; SAT subject exams recommended but not required in one or more of math (level 2), biology, chemistry, and literature

ACT

31

2010–2011 ACCEPTANCES

	In State	Out of State	Total
Applicants			
Interviewed			
New students			

No information provided

FACTORS REQUIRED TO CONTINUE IN PROGRAM

3.5 GPA each semester; science GPA after three years must be at least 3.5.

MCAT REQUIRED

Yes, minimum score 29 with no subsection score lower than 7

FINANCIAL AID

No special financial aid for students in the program

COST

	Resident Tuition and Fees ($)	Non Resident Tuition and Fees ($)
Undergraduate	5970	not applicable
Medical school	28,555	not applicable

COLLEGE
University of Miami

MEDICAL SCHOOL
University of Miami Miller School of Medicine

ADDRESS
Office of Admissions
University of Miami
PO Box 248025
Coral Gables, Florida 33124-8025
305-284-4323
www.miami.edu/admission/index.php/undergraduate_admission
/academics/dual_degree_honors/honors_program_in_medicine/

NAME OF PROGRAM
Honors Program in Medicine

LENGTH OF PROGRAM
7 or 8 years

APPLICATION DEADLINE
November 1

INFORMATION ABOUT THE PROGRAM
Personal factors—the student's maturity, common sense, empathy, interpersonal skills, freedom from parental influence, and compassion for others—are as important as academic factors in the admissions process. Of critical importance to the admissions process, the student must have self-initiated patient contact experiences.

All students in the program are required to participate in a professionalism experience each semester they are enrolled in the undergraduate program. These experiences might include volunteering at health-related facilities, biomedical research, participation in area service organizations, or study abroad.

Students in the program are required to complete all of the requirements for a major and are not allowed to apply to other medical schools without the permission of the school of medicine.

TRANSFER STUDENTS CONSIDERED
No

CITIZENSHIP REQUIREMENTS
U.S. citizen or permanent resident visa

MINIMUM REQUIRED FACTORS IN SELECTION

CLASSES

Four years of English, four years of math, one year of biology, and one year of chemistry

GPA

Unweighted GPA of at least 3.75

SAT

1,400 on critical reading and math; SAT subject exams in math and one science, with minimum score of 600 on each test

ACT

32

2010–2011 ACCEPTANCES

	In State	Out of State	Total
Applicants	84	143	227
Interviewed	27	59	86
New students	8	3	11

FACTORS REQUIRED TO CONTINUE IN PROGRAM

Overall and science GPA of 3.7 and MCAT score of at least 30

MCAT REQUIRED

Yes, minimum score 30

FINANCIAL AID

No special financial aid for students in the program

COST

	Resident Tuition and Fees ($)	Non Resident Tuition and Fees ($)
Undergraduate	41,220	41,220
Medical school	32,672	42,154

COLLEGE

University of Hawai'i at Manoa

MEDICAL SCHOOL

John A. Burns School of Medicine

ADDRESS

University of Hawai'i at Manoa
Office of Admissions
2600 Campus Road, Room 001
Honolulu, Hawai'i 96822-2385
808-956-8975
www.manoa.hawaii.edu/admissions/undergrad/early_admissions/

NAME OF PROGRAM

Doctor of Medicine Early Acceptance Program

LENGTH OF PROGRAM

8 years

APPLICATION DEADLINE

January 5

INFORMATION ABOUT THE PROGRAM

This is a new program that is in the process of being established. Students in the program will be part of the honors program at the college and will participate in summer clinical, research, and service internships. Volunteering and physician shadowing are part of the program requirements.

Students will also have early interaction with faculty from the medical school. There are several study abroad programs available for students in the program, and fourth year medical students will have the opportunity for medical study abroad.

There are two applications required, including application to the college and application to the program. A supplemental essay, letters of recommendation, and résumé are also required as part of the application.

TRANSFER STUDENTS CONSIDERED

No

CITIZENSHIP REQUIREMENTS

U.S. citizen or permanent resident visa. Must also be a resident of Hawai'i.

MINIMUM REQUIRED FACTORS IN SELECTION

CLASSES

Pre-calculus, biology, chemistry, and physics must be completed or in progress. Students are expected to have AP credits.

GPA

Unweighted GPA of at least 3.8

SAT

1,800

ACT

27

2010–2011 ACCEPTANCES

	In State	Out of State	Total
Applicants			
Interviewed			
New students			

New program; no information exists for previous years

FACTORS REQUIRED TO CONTINUE IN PROGRAM

3.5 cumulative GPA and 3.4 science GPA; maintain full-time status in the honors program

MCAT REQUIRED

Yes, minimum score of 30 with minimum 9 in any section or 31 with minimum of 8 in any section

FINANCIAL AID

Undergraduate tuition covers all four years of undergraduate education for students in the program.

COST

	Resident Tuition and Fees ($)	Non Resident Tuition and Fees ($)
Undergraduate	0	not applicable
Medical school	30,742	not applicable

COLLEGE

Northwestern University

MEDICAL SCHOOL

Northwestern University Feinberg School of Medicine

ADDRESS

Associate Dean for Medical Education

Office of Admission and Financial Aid Northwestern University

1801 Hinman Avenue

Evanston, Illinois 60204-3060

312-503-8915

www.feinberg.northwestern.edu/AWOME/hpme/

NAME OF PROGRAM

Honors Program in Medical Education (HPME)

LENGTH OF PROGRAM

7 or 8 years

APPLICATION DEADLINE

December 1 for request for HPME application; January 1 for submission of application

INFORMATION ABOUT THE PROGRAM

Although often listed as a seven-year program, HPME encourages its students to consider spending eight years in the program. The goal of the program is to train the best students for a career in medicine while reducing the stress often associated with medical school applications. Students are encouraged to challenge themselves during their undergraduate years in an effort to develop personally and professionally.

As undergraduates, students may attend the Weinberg College of Arts, the School of Communication, or the McCormick School of Engineering at Northwestern. The courses they take depend on which undergraduate school they attend.

Students are provided with regular counseling to discuss the various options to them as undergraduates. There is a strong mentoring program available as part of the HPME program. There are also programs available where students can earn a PhD or a master's in public health (MPH). A summer research program is available to interested students after the first year of medical school.

This is a non-binding program and students are allowed to apply to other medical schools.

TRANSFER STUDENTS CONSIDERED

No

CITIZENSHIP REQUIREMENTS
International students accepted

MINIMUM REQUIRED FACTORS IN SELECTION

CLASSES
Four years of math (one year of calculus including differential and integral calculus are required before beginning HPME; if this is not offered at your high school, you must take the course before entering Northwestern); one year of chemistry; one year of physics; one year of biology; four years of English; two years of foreign language (three to four years of the same language preferred)

GPA
No minimum but students are typically in top five percent of high school class

SAT
No minimum, but averages for accepted students are critical reading, 762; math, 770; writing, 770; subject tests in chemistry and math level 2 are required; no minimum, but averages for accepted students are chemistry, 762; and math level 2, 775

ACT
No minimum, but average is 34

2010–2011 ACCEPTANCES

	In State	Out of State	Total
Applicants	96	521	617
Interviewed			
New students	6	25	31

FACTORS REQUIRED TO CONTINUE IN PROGRAM
Students are required to have a minimum 3.2 GPA in sciences courses and a minimum 3.4 GPA in overall academic courses.

MCAT REQUIRED
No

FINANCIAL AID
Northwestern meets one hundred percent of the demonstrated need for a student's undergraduate education. Northwestern also has financial aid available for medical school students.

COST

	Resident Tuition and Fees ($)	Non Resident Tuition and Fees ($)
Undergraduate	43,380	43,380
Medical school	48,339	48,449

COLLEGE

University of Illinois at Chicago

MEDICAL SCHOOL

University of Illinois at Chicago College of Medicine

ADDRESS

Assistant Director Academic Affairs/
Special Scholarship Programs
University of Illinois at Chicago
2506 University Hall, M/C 115
601 S. Morgan Street
Chicago, Illinois 60607-7100
312-355-2477
www.uic.edu/depts/oaa/spec_prog/gppa/gppamedicine/

NAME OF PROGRAM

Guaranteed Professional Programs Admissions (GPPA)

LENGTH OF PROGRAM

8 years

APPLICATION DEADLINE

December 1

INFORMATION ABOUT THE PROGRAM

Students in this program are also expected to apply to and participate in the Honors College of the university. This provides some
advantages in the way of services and facilities. An honors college interview is required. Students are allowed to major in any
subject offered by the university's eight undergraduate colleges.
While in the program, students must complete an independent
study project, which includes a presentation. There are several
professionalism courses offered by the college of medicine that students are required to attend.

The program places special emphasis on professionalism, integrity, and compassion for the human spirit.

Students may apply to medical schools outside the program.

TRANSFER STUDENTS CONSIDERED

No

CITIZENSHIP REQUIREMENTS

U.S. citizen or permanent resident visa; must also be Illinois
resident

MINIMUM REQUIRED FACTORS IN SELECTION

CLASSES

No specific requirement

GPA

Top fifteen percent of high school class. Average admitted student was in the top two percent of high school class.

SAT

1,240 critical reading and math

ACT

28; average admitted score was approximately 33.

2011–2012 ACCEPTANCES

	In State	Out of State	Total
Applicants	400±		400±
Interviewed	100±		100±
New students	20 to 25		20 to 25

FACTORS REQUIRED TO CONTINUE IN PROGRAM

3.5 GPA, maintaining status in the Honors College, completion of required courses related to the medical profession, and completion of an independent study seminar project and presentation

MCAT REQUIRED

Yes; must earn score of at least the mean of the matriculating students into the College of Medicine in the year prior to expected entry, with no score below 9 for any segment of the exam.

FINANCIAL AID

In addition to regular financial aid, students admitted to the program are also considered for the Chancellor's GPPA Excellence Award of tuition and a portion of fees, renewable for the four years of undergraduate college.

COST

	Resident Tuition and Fees ($)	Non Resident Tuition and Fees ($)
Undergraduate	13,463	not applicable
Medical school	35,344	not applicable

COLLEGE
Indiana State University

MEDICAL SCHOOL
Indiana University School of Medicine

ADDRESS
Stalker Hall 214
Indiana State University
200 North Seventh Street
Terre Haute, Indiana 47809-9989
812-237-8633
www.indstate.edu/preprof/rhp.htm

NAME OF PROGRAM
B/MD Rural Health Program

LENGTH OF PROGRAM
8 years

APPLICATION DEADLINE
November 15

INFORMATION ABOUT THE PROGRAM
This specialized program is only open to residents of rural Indiana. Students may major in any undergraduate degree. Students in the program have interaction with faculty of the school of medicine including the opportunity to participate in a mini-medical school. Students also have summer internship experiences with rural physicians and undergraduate research experience.

TRANSFER STUDENTS CONSIDERED
No

CITIZENSHIP REQUIREMENTS
U.S. citizen or permanent resident visa; must reside in rural Indiana

MINIMUM REQUIRED FACTORS IN SELECTION

CLASSES

No specific requirement

GPA

3.5

SAT

1,200 critical reading and math

ACT

27

2011–2012 ACCEPTANCES

	In State	Out of State	Total
Applicants			
Interviewed			
New students			9

No information provided

FACTORS REQUIRED TO CONTINUE IN PROGRAM

Undergraduate minimum GPA of 3.5

MCAT REQUIRED

Yes; score must be at least equal to the mean score of the previous year's entering class.

FINANCIAL AID

Students in program receive full tuition waiver for undergraduate study.

COST

	Resident Tuition and Fees ($)	Non Resident Tuition and Fees ($)
Undergraduate	0	not applicable
Medical school	33,146	not applicable

COLLEGE
University of Kentucky

MEDICAL SCHOOL
University of Kentucky College of Medicine

ADDRESS
University of Kentucky
Undergraduate Admissions
100 W. D. Funkhouser Building
Lexington, Kentucky 40506-0054
www.mc.uky.edu/meded/bsmd/

NAME OF PROGRAM
B.S./M.D. Accelerated Course of Study Program

LENGTH OF PROGRAM
7 years

APPLICATION DEADLINE
January 15. This date varies by a few days each year.

INFORMATION ABOUT THE PROGRAM
Students have to complete three applications including an undergraduate application, an application to the Academic Scholarship Program and a B.S./M.D. Admission Application. There is also a supplemental essay describing your background, why you wish to be a physician and why you are interested in the university. Students must declare a major in biology. Students take the MCAT after their second undergraduate year.

Technically, this is an early assurance type program, but on average about ninety percent of the students in the program do advance to the medical school.

TRANSFER STUDENTS CONSIDERED
No

CITIZENSHIP REQUIREMENTS
U.S. citizen or permanent resident visa

CLASSES

AP classes in biology and chemistry are recommended.

GPA

Unweighted GPA of at least 3.5

SAT

1,360 critical reading and math

ACT

31

2010–2011 ACCEPTANCES

	In State	Out of State	Total
Applicants			
Interviewed			
New students			5–10

No information provided

FACTORS REQUIRED TO CONTINUE IN PROGRAM

3.5 overall GPA

MCAT REQUIRED

Yes; no minimum defined but must be exceptional

FINANCIAL AID

No special financial aid for students in the program

COST

	Resident Tuition and Fees ($)	Non Resident Tuition and Fees ($)
Undergraduate	9,676	19,864
Medical school	32,889	60,334

COLLEGE
University of Louisville

MEDICAL SCHOOL
University of Louisville School of Medicine

ADDRESS
Office of Admissions
University of Louisville
Houchens Building, Room 150
2211 S. Brook Street
Louisville, Kentucky 40208-1874
502-852-6531
https://louisville.edu/admissions/aid/gep/gems

NAME OF PROGRAM
Guaranteed Entrance to Medical School (GEMS)

LENGTH OF PROGRAM
8 years

APPLICATION DEADLINE
February 15

INFORMATION ABOUT THE PROGRAM
Students in the program will have hands-on experience with the medical school, including physician shadowing and enhanced opportunities for research and professional meetings. Applicants to the program need to provide an essay discussing their plans and goals for the future; three recommendation letters, including one from a principal or counselor, one from a science or math teacher, and a third from another non-high school, non-family member adult who knows the student.

TRANSFER STUDENTS CONSIDERED
No

CITIZENSHIP REQUIREMENTS
U.S. citizen or permanent resident visa; must also be a resident of Kentucky and attend high school in Kentucky

MINIMUM REQUIRED FACTORS IN SELECTION

CLASSES

No specific requirement

GPA

Unweighted GPA of at least 3.75; top five percent of high school class

SAT

1,330 critical reading and math

ACT

30

2010–2011 ACCEPTANCES

	In State	Out of State	Total
Applicants			
Interviewed			
New students	7		7

No information provided

FACTORS REQUIRED TO CONTINUE IN PROGRAM

3.4 cumulative GPA

MCAT REQUIRED

Yes; score at or above the national mean on each section of the test

FINANCIAL AID

No special financial aid for students in the program

COST

	Resident Tuition and Fees ($)	Non Resident Tuition and Fees ($)
Undergraduate	9,466	not applicable
Medical school	31,512	not applicable

COLLEGE
Boston University

MEDICAL SCHOOL
Boston University School of Medicine

ADDRESS
Boston University
Office of Undergraduate Admissions
121 Bay State Road
Boston, Massachusetts 02215-1714
617-353-2300
www.bu.edu/academics/cas/programs
/seven-year-liberal-arts-medical-education-program/

NAME OF PROGRAM
Seven-Year Program of Liberal Arts and Medical Education

LENGTH OF PROGRAM
7 years

APPLICATION DEADLINE
November 15

INFORMATION ABOUT THE PROGRAM
Students spend the first three years of the program studying at the College of Arts & Sciences. During this time they take premedical science courses as well as elective course in the humanities and social sciences. Students are also required to take a biology course and other elective courses during the second summer in the program. After completing the required undergraduate science courses in the first two years of the program, students may take modular medical courses in the third year of the program. Many of these modular courses are equivalent to first year medical school courses.

All students are also required to complete a minor in a discipline approved by the College of Arts & Sciences. Students are not allowed to apply to other medical schools and remain in the program.

TRANSFER STUDENTS CONSIDERED
No

CITIZENSHIP REQUIREMENTS
International students considered

MINIMUM REQUIRED FACTORS IN SELECTION

CLASSES

Four years English and math including one year of calculus, three years social sciences, three years foreign languages, one year biology, one year physics, one year of chemistry (AP chemistry recommended)

GPA

No specific GPA; typical successful applicants had a 3.9 GPA unweighted and were in the top one percent of their high school class.

SAT

No specific SAT; average SAT score of successful candidates was 2,266; subject tests are required in math level 2 and chemistry; subject test in a foreign language is recommended; average chemistry subject test score, 757; average math level 2 score, 779.

ACT

No specific requirement

2011–2012 ACCEPTANCES

	In State	Out of State	Total
Applicants	62	669	730
Interviewed	2	94	96
New students	1	20	21

FACTORS REQUIRED TO CONTINUE IN PROGRAM

3.2 GPA cumulative and in the sciences

MCAT REQUIRED

Yes; minimum score of 30

FINANCIAL AID

Need-based aid available for undergraduates; loans available for medical school students

COST

	Resident Tuition and Fees ($)	Non Resident Tuition and Fees ($)
Undergraduate	42,994	42,994
Medical school	50,948	50,948

COLLEGE

Michigan Technological University

MEDICAL SCHOOL

Wayne State University School of Medicine

ADDRESS

Department of Biological Sciences
Michigan Technological University
1400 Townsend Drive
Houghton, Michigan 49931-1295
906-487-2335
www.admissions.mtu.edu/medstart/

NAME OF PROGRAM

WSU MedStart at Michigan Tech

LENGTH OF PROGRAM

8 years

APPLICATION DEADLINE

February 1

INFORMATION ABOUT THE PROGRAM

The program emphasizes mentoring and research activities and includes early contact with faculty and students of the medical school. The program is designed to train future medical innovators and creative thinkers.

TRANSFER STUDENTS CONSIDERED

No

CITIZENSHIP REQUIREMENTS

U.S. citizen or permanent resident visa; Canadian residents also considered

MINIMUM REQUIRED FACTORS IN SELECTION

CLASSES

No specific requirement

GPA

3.5 unweighted GPA

SAT

No specific requirement

ACT

25

2010–2011 ACCEPTANCES

	In State	Out of State	Total
Applicants			
Interviewed			
New students			2

FACTORS REQUIRED TO CONTINUE IN PROGRAM

Must maintain a 3.3 unweighted GPA; must complete required science courses and an English composition course with grades of B or better; must participate in the WSU MedStart at Michigan Tech seminar and continue involvement with medical volunteer work

MCAT REQUIRED

Yes; minimum score 30

FINANCIAL AID

COST

	Resident Tuition and Fees ($)	Non Resident Tuition and Fees ($)
Undergraduate	13,353	27,258
Medical school	32,198	64,898

COLLEGE

Northern Michigan University

MEDICAL SCHOOL

Wayne State University School of Medicine

ADDRESS

Director of Admissions
Northern Michigan University
1401 Presque Isle Avenue
Marquette, Michigan 49855-5305
906-227-2650
http://webb.nmu.edu/Programs/PreProfessional/SiteSections
/MedStart/MedStart.shtml

NAME OF PROGRAM

MedStart

LENGTH OF PROGRAM

8 years

APPLICATION DEADLINE

February 1

INFORMATION ABOUT THE PROGRAM

The program emphasizes mentoring and research activities and
includes early contact with faculty and students of the medical
school. A number of activities are available for students in the pre-
medical program at Northern Michigan University; students are
expected to take advantage of the opportunities, including pre-
professional clubs and hospital seminars.

Preference in admissions is given to students from medically
underserved areas who have an interest in working as a primary
care physician in such areas.

TRANSFER STUDENTS CONSIDERED

No

CITIZENSHIP REQUIREMENTS

U.S. citizen or permanent resident visa

MINIMUM REQUIRED FACTORS IN SELECTION

CLASSES
No specific requirement

GPA
3.5 in academic core courses; classes are weighted for AP/IB/honors courses

SAT
1,240 on critical reading and math

ACT
28

2010–2011 ACCEPTANCES

	In State	Out of State	Total
Applicants			
Interviewed			
New students			2

FACTORS REQUIRED TO CONTINUE IN PROGRAM
Cumulative GPA of 3.3 and active participation in the college's premedical activities; ongoing involvement with health-related volunteer work

MCAT REQUIRED
Yes; minimum score 24 with at least an 8 in biological sciences

FINANCIAL AID
Students in the program are guaranteed scholarship support at the college.

COST

	Resident Tuition and Fees ($)	Non Resident Tuition and Fees ($)
Undergraduate	8,646	13,542
Medical school	32,198	64,898

COLLEGE
Wayne State University

MEDICAL SCHOOL
Wayne State University School of Medicine

ADDRESS
Program Coordinator
Irvin D. Reid Honors College
Wayne State University
2100 Undergraduate Library
Detroit, Michigan 48202-3900
313-577-8523
www.honors.wayne.edu/medstart.php

NAME OF PROGRAM
Medstart

LENGTH OF PROGRAM
8 years

APPLICATION DEADLINE
November 15

INFORMATION ABOUT THE PROGRAM
Students applying to the program must have admissions to Wayne State University by November 15. A separate application to the program along with all other documentation must be completed by January 1.

The program emphasizes mentoring and research activities and includes early contact with faculty and students of the medical school. A number of activities are available for students in the program, and students are expected to take advantage of the opportunities. These include participation in the university's branch of American Medical Student Association and participation in information and recruitment sessions for new students.

TRANSFER STUDENTS CONSIDERED
No

CITIZENSHIP REQUIREMENTS
U.S. citizen or permanent resident visa; Canadian citizens also considered

MINIMUM REQUIRED FACTORS IN SELECTION

CLASSES
No specific requirement

GPA
3.75

SAT
2,010

ACT
30

2011–2012 ACCEPTANCES

	In State	Out of State	Total
Applicants	202	99	301
Interviewed	30	6	36
New students	14	1	15

FACTORS REQUIRED TO CONTINUE IN PROGRAM
Good standing in the honors college with a 3.3 GPA for the first year and a 3.5 GPA thereafter; 3.5 GPA in biology, chemistry, physics, and math, with no grade less than a B; participation in MedStart seminars, physician shadowing experiences, volunteer work in a health care field, and various aspects of the MedStart program. Students must apply for an undergraduate research grant prior to senior year and graduate with university honors, including a senior thesis and senior seminar.

MCAT REQUIRED
Yes; 10 on each section and minimum total of 30.

FINANCIAL AID
Students admitted to MedStart are provided a scholarship.

COST

	Resident Tuition and Fees ($)	Non Resident Tuition and Fees ($)
Undergraduate	10,190	21,735
Medical school	32,198	64,898

COLLEGE

St. Louis University

MEDICAL SCHOOL

St. Louis University School of Medicine

ADDRESS

Preprofessional Health Studies
Verhaegen Hall, Room 314
3634 Lindell Boulevard
St. Louis, Missouri 63108-3302
314-977-2840
www.slu.edu/x24610.xml

NAME OF PROGRAM

Medical Scholars Program

LENGTH OF PROGRAM

8 years

APPLICATION DEADLINE

December 1

INFORMATION ABOUT THE PROGRAM

Technically, this is not a true BS/MD program with guaranteed admission to medical school from high school. Instead, scholars are selected for the medical school track while they are in high school; the actual medical school application occurs the spring semester of sophomore year in college. However, medical scholars do have a ninety-eight percent acceptance rate into the medical school; so I have included this program with the traditional programs, since the effect is basically the same.

Freshmen in the program take a medical scholars seminar their spring semester. All medical scholars must complete at least one math course at the college. Students in the program who apply to other medical schools will have their early acceptance withdrawn.

TRANSFER STUDENTS CONSIDERED

No

CITIZENSHIP REQUIREMENTS

International students considered

MINIMUM REQUIRED FACTORS IN SELECTION

CLASSES

One year of biology, one year of chemistry, and three years of math

GPA

No minimum, but typical selected candidates rank in the top ten percent of their high school class

SAT

1,330 critical reading and math

ACT

30

2010–2011 ACCEPTANCES

	In State	Out of State	Total
Applicants	121	430	551
Interviewed			
New students	30	101	131

FACTORS REQUIRED TO CONTINUE IN PROGRAM

Minimum 3.4 cumulative GPA and 3.4 science and math GPA after freshman year. Minimum 3.5 cumulative GPA and 3.5 science and math GPA for other undergraduate years.

MCAT REQUIRED

Yes; no minimum score required

FINANCIAL AID

COST

	Resident Tuition and Fees ($)	Non Resident Tuition and Fees ($)
Undergraduate	35,246	35,246
Medical school	48,130	48,130

COLLEGE
University of Missouri Kansas City

MEDICAL SCHOOL
University of Missouri Kansas City School of Medicine

ADDRESS
UMKC School of Medicine
Council on Selection
2411 Holmes
Kansas City, Missouri 64108-2792
816-235-1870
www.med.umkc.edu/med_admissions/BAMD.shtml

NAME OF PROGRAM
Six Year B.A./M.D. Program

LENGTH OF PROGRAM
6 years

APPLICATION DEADLINE
November 1

INFORMATION ABOUT THE PROGRAM
This program is one of the largest in the country. The majority of
students in the medical school come through the BA/MD program.
This is a year-round program; and the medical school classes and
undergraduate classes are combined during all six years.

During the first two years of the program, three quarters of
the student's time is spent on the arts and science education required to fulfill the BA degree requirements; one quarter of the
time is spent on medical school courses. During this time students
are assigned primary care physicians to mentor the students in
the fundamentals of medicine. During the last four years of the
program this ratio is reversed, with three quarters of the time
spent on medical school courses and one quarter of the time on
courses to fulfill the BA degree requirements.

There is an emphasis on medical humanities at the school of
medicine; and during year five or six the student spends a month
gaining a broader appreciation of art, literature, and philosophy,
while cultivating compassion and empathy.

During years three to six, the student is assigned to a docent
unit, which also includes a senior student, a clinical pharmacolo-
gist, and other health care professionals. These units provide a
small group learning environment, and each unit spends a half
day per week providing outpatient care in local clinics.

Fifth year students spend one month in a rural Missouri preceptorship to provide experience in addressing health care con-

cerns in a non-urban primary care clinic as well as experience with the business operation of a small town physician.

TRANSFER STUDENTS CONSIDERED

Yes, for students with fewer than twenty-four hours of post–high school college credit

CITIZENSHIP REQUIREMENTS

U.S. citizen or permanent resident visa; students must also have graduated from a U.S. accredited high school

MINIMUM REQUIRED FACTORS IN SELECTION

CLASSES

Four years of English and math, three years of science (including one year of biology and one year of chemistry), two years of a single foreign language, and one year of fine arts

GPA

3.0; average GPA of accepted Missouri residents is 3.80 and of out-of-state residents is 3.85

SAT

1,030. Accepted for out-of-state residents but ACT preferred; average for out-of-state residents is 1,380.

ACT

22. ACT required for Missouri residents; average ACT for accepted in-state residents is 30; average for out-of-state residents is 31

2011–2012 ACCEPTANCES

	In State	Out of State	Total
Applicants	291	542	833
Interviewed	134	164	298
New students	62	51	113

FACTORS REQUIRED TO CONTINUE IN PROGRAM

Minimum cumulative 2.7 GPA

MCAT REQUIRED

No

FINANCIAL AID

No special financial aid for students in the program

COST

	Resident Tuition and Fees ($)	Non Resident Tuition and Fees ($)
Undergraduate	13,706	32,507
Medical school	27,814	48,588

COLLEGE
Washington University in St. Louis

MEDICAL SCHOOL
Washington University in St. Louis School of Medicine

ADDRESS
Undergraduate Admissions
Washington University in St. Louis
One Brookings Drive
St. Louis, Missouri 63130-4862
314-935-6000
http://admissions.wustl.edu/usp/Pages/default.aspx

NAME OF PROGRAM
University Scholars Program in Medicine

LENGTH OF PROGRAM
8 years

APPLICATION DEADLINE
January 15

INFORMATION ABOUT THE PROGRAM
Students may major in any subject. Students are welcome to engage in study abroad programs. Students in the program often engage in research if they desire, and this is often with faculty members of the medical school. Program participants have the opportunity for doctor shadowing and personalized pre-professional advising. Students in the program are allowed to apply to other medical schools.

Students considering this program should be aware of several factors. The requirements for students to advance to the medical school are the most stringent of any BS/MD program. Participants are required to maintain a high GPA and have a very high MCAT score. It is also my experience that for admittance to the program, students should show particular interest in Washington University, including visiting the campus if at all possible.

TRANSFER STUDENTS CONSIDERED
No

CITIZENSHIP REQUIREMENTS
International students considered

MINIMUM REQUIRED FACTORS IN SELECTION

None specified

2010–2011 ACCEPTANCES

	In State	Out of State	Total
Applicants			380
Interviewed			
New students			10

FACTORS REQUIRED TO CONTINUE IN PROGRAM

3.8 GPA overall

MCAT REQUIRED

Yes; minimum score of 36 required

FINANCIAL AID

There are no scholarships specified for students in the program. Washington University does meet one hundred percent of the need of admitted students for undergraduate study. The medical school does have need-based scholarships and loans. There are also merit-based scholarships available for the medical school.

COST

	Resident Tuition and Fees ($)	Non Resident Tuition and Fees ($)
Undergraduate	42,925	42,925
Medical school	50,510	50,510

COLLEGE
Chadron State College; Wayne State College

MEDICAL SCHOOL
University of Nebraska Medical Center

ADDRESS
Health Professions Office
Chadron State College
1000 Main Street
Chadron, Nebraska 69337
308-432-6278
www.csc.edu/sci/rhop/

Health Professions Office
Wayne State College
1111 Main Street
Wayne, Nebraska 68787
402-375-7329
www.wsc.edu/schools/nss/rhop/

NAME OF PROGRAM
Rural Health Opportunities Program

LENGTH OF PROGRAM
8 years

APPLICATION DEADLINE
December 1

INFORMATION ABOUT THE PROGRAM
The purpose of this program is to educate students from rural Nebraska who wish to return to practice medicine in rural areas of the state. Students may apply to only one of the programs, not both.

TRANSFER STUDENTS CONSIDERED
No

CITIZENSHIP REQUIREMENTS
U.S. citizen or permanent resident visa; must be a resident of rural Nebraska and a graduate of a Nebraska high school

MINIMUM REQUIRED FACTORS IN SELECTION

CLASSES

Strongly recommend four years of English, three years of math, and one year each of biology, chemistry, and physics

GPA

No specific requirement

SAT

No specific requirement

ACT

No specific requirement

2010–2011 ACCEPTANCES

	In State	Out of State	Total
Applicants	70 Chadron 60 Wayne		
Interviewed	35 Chadron 20 Wayne		
New students	29 Chadron 5 Wayne		

FACTORS REQUIRED TO CONTINUE IN PROGRAM

3.5 overall and a C or better in every class

MCAT REQUIRED

Yes; minimum score 24

FINANCIAL AID

Students in the program will receive tuition waiver for up to sixteen credits per term during their undergraduate years.

COST

	Resident Tuition and Fees ($)	Non Resident Tuition and Fees ($)
Undergraduate	0	not applicable
Medical school	27,992	not applicable

COLLEGE
University of Nevada, Las Vegas; University of Nevada, Reno

MEDICAL SCHOOL
University of Nevada School of Medicine

ADDRESS
University of Nevada School of Medicine
Mailstop 0357-Pennington Medical Education Building
Reno, Nevada 89557-0357
775-784-6063
www.medicine.nevada.edu/dept/asa/prospective_applicants
/programs_bsmd.htm

NAME OF PROGRAM
BS-MD Accelerated Early Admission Program

LENGTH OF PROGRAM
7 years

APPLICATION DEADLINE
February 25

INFORMATION ABOUT THE PROGRAM
Each of the undergraduate colleges associated with this program
may have up to six students admitted into the program. Students
must select which college they wish to apply to before applying to
the program. Research and clinical experience is expected of all
students in the program during their undergraduate years.

TRANSFER STUDENTS CONSIDERED
No

CITIZENSHIP REQUIREMENTS
U.S. citizen or permanent resident visa; Nevada residency; must
also attend a Nevada high school for a minimum of two years and
graduate from a Nevada high school

MINIMUM REQUIRED FACTORS IN SELECTION

CLASSES

No specific requirement

GPA

3.7 unweighted or top ten percent of high school class

SAT

1,270 on critical reading and math

ACT

29

2010–2011 ACCEPTANCES

	In State	Out of State	Total
Applicants	35	0	35
Interviewed	28	0	28
New students	12	0	12

FACTORS REQUIRED TO CONTINUE IN PROGRAM

3.5 overall and science GPA

MCAT REQUIRED

Yes; minimum score 28 with no sub-score below 7

FINANCIAL AID

No special financial aid for students in the program

COST

	Resident Tuition and Fees ($)	Non Resident Tuition and Fees ($)
Undergraduate	6,793	not applicable
Medical school	20,700	not applicable

COLLEGE

Caldwell College

MEDICAL SCHOOL

New Jersey Medical School

ADDRESS

Caldwell College
120 Bloomfield Avenue
Caldwell, New Jersey 07006-5310
973-618-3000
www.caldwell.edu/health-professionals/Affiliation.aspx

NAME OF PROGRAM

Health Professions Affiliation Program Medicine

LENGTH OF PROGRAM

7 or 8 years

APPLICATION DEADLINE

January 15

INFORMATION ABOUT THE PROGRAM

This is one of eight programs associated with the New Jersey
Medical School. Students can major in any topic.

TRANSFER STUDENTS CONSIDERED

No

CITIZENSHIP REQUIREMENTS

U.S. citizen or permanent resident visa

MINIMUM REQUIRED FACTORS IN SELECTION

CLASSES

No specific requirements

GPA

3.50 unweighted

SAT

1,400 critical reading and math

ACT

32

2011–2012 ACCEPTANCES

	In State	Out of State	Total
Applicants			400
Interviewed			80
New students			20

Note: these numbers reflect applications and admissions for all eight programs associated with New Jersey Medical School.

FACTORS REQUIRED TO CONTINUE IN PROGRAM

No information provided

MCAT REQUIRED

No information provided.

FINANCIAL AID

No special financial aid for students in the program

COST

	Resident Tuition and Fees ($)	Non Resident Tuition and Fees ($)
Undergraduate	28,185	28,185
Medical school	38,550	38,550

COLLEGE
The College of New Jersey

MEDICAL SCHOOL
New Jersey Medical School

ADDRESS
Chairman, Medical Careers Committee
The College of New Jersey
PO Box 7718
Ewing, New Jersey 08628-0718
609-771-2021
www.tcnj.edu/~biology/7med/medfaq.html

NAME OF PROGRAM
Combined BS/MD 7-Year Program

LENGTH OF PROGRAM
7 years

APPLICATION DEADLINE
December 1

INFORMATION ABOUT THE PROGRAM
This is one of eight programs associated with the New Jersey Medical School. Students in the program spend three years at the college and must major in an approved major—biology, chemistry, English, philosophy, biomedical engineering, math, economics, physics, or history. No additional time is required at the college other than a summer research project that must be completed before the first year of medical school.

Students with high academic achievement and a record of community service may be asked to interview with a medical career advisor at the college. Telephone interviews are allowed only for students living far from New Jersey. If that interview is favorable you will then be asked to interview with the medical school admissions office at the medical school. This interview must be in person. Typically, half of the students in the eight BS/MD programs associated with New Jersey Medical School come from The College of New Jersey. Students in the program are allowed to apply out to other medical schools during the fourth year of the program, but they will then lose their guaranteed acceptance to the medical school.

TRANSFER STUDENTS CONSIDERED
No

CITIZENSHIP REQUIREMENTS
U.S. citizen or permanent resident visa. Students who do not have U.S. citizenship or permanent resident status may apply as long

as they qualify for citizenship or permanent resident status before starting at the medical school.

MINIMUM REQUIRED FACTORS IN SELECTION

CLASSES

No specific requirement

GPA

Top five percent or have a GPA of 4.5 or 95 percent, depending on the school. If high school does not rank, the admissions office will call the head guidance counselor of your school to evaluate your ranking and transcript. Average GPA of accepted students is 4.72.

SAT

1,480 critical reading and math. Average score of accepted students is 1,534. SAT subject tests are optional, but of those submitted, the average score was 773.

ACT

Not accepted

2011–2012 ACCEPTANCES

	In State	Out of State	Total
Applicants			400
Interviewed			80
New students			20

Note: these numbers reflect applications and admissions for all eight programs associated with New Jersey Medical School.

FACTORS REQUIRED TO CONTINUE IN PROGRAM

3.5 cumulative and science GPA in approved major; grade of B or better in each of the basic science courses required by the medical school; no grade below a C in any course. Students must engage in a research experience before beginning the medical school.

MCAT REQUIRED

Yes; no minimum score required, but students are encouraged to achieve at least a 31.

FINANCIAL AID

No special financial aid for students in the program

COST

	Resident Tuition and Fees ($)	Non Resident Tuition and Fees ($)
Undergraduate	14,702	24,854
Medical school	38,550	38,550

COLLEGE
Drew University

MEDICAL SCHOOL
New Jersey Medical School

ADDRESS
College Admissions
Drew University
36 Madison Avenue
Madison, New Jersey 07940-1434
973-408-3739
www.drew.edu/undergraduate/what-you-learn/pre-med/
dual-degree

NAME OF PROGRAM
Dual-Degree Program (B.A./M.D.) in Medicine

LENGTH OF PROGRAM
7 years

APPLICATION DEADLINE
December 1

INFORMATION ABOUT THE PROGRAM
This is one of eight programs associated with the New Jersey
Medical School. Students in the program may major in any subject
while at Drew. In addition to major requirements, a student must
meet general education requirements and take basic pre-medical
courses. Drew typically receives 60 to 100 applications to this program and 10 to 20 of these are accepted into the medical school.

An in-person interview with Drew University is required and
should be held by December 1. The applications of qualified candidates will then be sent to the medical school, where students will
be selected for in-person interviews at the medical school. A student may apply to other medical schools but will lose their guaranteed spot if they do so.

TRANSFER STUDENTS CONSIDERED
No

CITIZENSHIP REQUIREMENTS
U.S. citizen or permanent resident visa

MINIMUM REQUIRED FACTORS IN SELECTION

CLASSES

No specific requirement

GPA

Top ten percent of high school class

SAT

1,400 critical reading and math

ACT

32

2011–2012 ACCEPTANCES

	In State	Out of State	Total
Applicants			400
Interviewed			80
New students			20

Note: these numbers reflect applications and admissions for all eight programs associated with New Jersey Medical School.

FACTORS REQUIRED TO CONTINUE IN PROGRAM

Students must carry at least fourteen credit hours per semester and maintain a 3.4 GPA overall and for science courses. No grade lower than a B– is allowed in one of the required pre-medical courses.

MCAT REQUIRED

Yes; no minimum score required

FINANCIAL AID

No special financial aid for students in the program

COST

	Resident Tuition and Fees ($)	Non Resident Tuition and Fees ($)
Undergraduate	47,510	47,510
Medical school	38,550	38,550

COLLEGE
Montclair State University

MEDICAL SCHOOL
New Jersey Medical School

ADDRESS
Health Professions Committee
Department of Biology
Montclair State University
1 Normal Avenue
Montclair, New Jersey 07043-1699
973-655-4397
www.montclair.edu/csam/health-careers/combined-bs-md/

NAME OF PROGRAM
Eight Year Combined BS/MD Program

LENGTH OF PROGRAM
8 years

APPLICATION DEADLINE
December 15

INFORMATION ABOUT THE PROGRAM
This is one of eight programs associated with the New Jersey
Medical School. This program is for students from financially and
educationally disadvantaged backgrounds. An in-person interview
at the college is offered to selected students. A parent or guardian
must accompany the student to the interview. The student must
show motivation, maturity, and an understanding of the demands
of the medical profession during the interview. All students must
participate in the honors program. Letters of recommendation are
required from a teacher of math, a teacher of science, and an English teacher. The program will accept a maximum of five letters of
recommendation. After the first interview, selected students are
invited to interview with the medical school.

TRANSFER STUDENTS CONSIDERED
No

CITIZENSHIP REQUIREMENTS
U.S. citizen or permanent resident visa and New Jersey resident

MINIMUM REQUIRED FACTORS IN SELECTION

CLASSES

Four years English, two years of the same foreign language, two years social studies, three years math through at least geometry, one year of biology with lab, one year of chemistry with lab.

GPA

Top ten percent high school class and B average or above GPA and at least a B average in math and science

SAT

1,100 with at least 550 on both critical reading and math on a single test

ACT

Not accepted

2011–2012 ACCEPTANCES

	In State	Out of State	Total
Applicants			400
Interviewed			80
New students			20

Note: these numbers reflect applications and admissions for all eight programs associated with New Jersey Medical School.

FACTORS REQUIRED TO CONTINUE IN PROGRAM

GPA of 3.2 or better, minimum grade of B in required pre-med science courses; fulfillment of requirements of the honors curriculum; and participation in summer study or independent research at New Jersey Medical School

MCAT REQUIRED

Yes; no minimum score required

FINANCIAL AID

No special financial aid program for students in the program

COST

	Resident Tuition and Fees ($)	Non Resident Tuition and Fees ($)
Undergraduate	11,057	not applicable
Medical school	38,550	not applicable

COLLEGE
New Jersey Institute of Technology

MEDICAL SCHOOL
New Jersey Medical School

ADDRESS
Honors College
New Jersey Institute of Technology
University Heights
Newark, New Jersey 07102-1982
973-642-7664
http://honors.njit.edu/admission/pre-health-law/health.php

NAME OF PROGRAM
Accelerated Medical Program

LENGTH OF PROGRAM
7 years

APPLICATION DEADLINE
November 1

INFORMATION ABOUT THE PROGRAM
This is one of eight programs associated with the New Jersey Medical School. Students applying to this program are first required to interview and be accepted into the Honors College. Those accepted into the Honors College then have their application sent to the medical school for review. Applicants are expected to show they have knowledge of the medical field through research or volunteer activities. The curriculum at the Honors College includes research and professional exploration.

TRANSFER STUDENTS CONSIDERED
No

CITIZENSHIP REQUIREMENTS
U.S. citizen or permanent resident visa by start of professional program

MINIMUM REQUIRED FACTORS IN SELECTION

CLASSES

No specific requirement

GPA

Top ten percent of high school class

SAT

1,400 critical reading and math in one sitting

ACT

32

2011–2012 ACCEPTANCES

	In State	Out of State	Total
Applicants			400
Interviewed			80
New students			20

Note: these numbers reflect applications and admissions for all eight programs associated with New Jersey Medical School.

FACTORS REQUIRED TO CONTINUE IN PROGRAM

Students must maintain a 3.4 GPA each semester in the program; minimum B grade in all required science courses

MCAT REQUIRED

Yes; no minimum score required

FINANCIAL AID

Students admitted to program receive a scholarship that covers the full cost of attendance.

COST

	Resident Tuition and Fees ($)	Non Resident Tuition and Fees ($)
Undergraduate	0	0
Medical school	38,550	38,550

COLLEGE
The Richard Stockton College of New Jersey

MEDICAL SCHOOL
New Jersey Medical School

ADDRESS
The Richard Stockton College of New Jersey
Jimmie Leeds Road
Pomona, New Jersey 08240-0088
609-642-7664
http://intraweb.stockton.edu/eyos/admissions_home/content
/images/2011docs/dual%20degree%20health%20info.pdf

NAME OF PROGRAM
Dual Degree Health Professions Program

LENGTH OF PROGRAM
7 years

APPLICATION DEADLINE
December 15

INFORMATION ABOUT THE PROGRAM
This is one of eight programs associated with the New Jersey
Medical School. There is a supplemental application required for
this program in addition to the regular application for admission.

TRANSFER STUDENTS CONSIDERED
No

CITIZENSHIP REQUIREMENTS
U.S. citizen or permanent resident visa

MINIMUM REQUIRED FACTORS IN SELECTION

CLASSES

Four years of English, three years of science, three years of math

GPA

Top ten percent of high school class

SAT

700 each in the critical reading and math sections from one test

ACT

Not accepted

2011–2012 ACCEPTANCES

	In State	Out of State	Total
Applicants			400
Interviewed			80
New students			20

Note: these numbers reflect applications and admissions for all eight programs associated with New Jersey Medical School.

FACTORS REQUIRED TO CONTINUE IN PROGRAM

Minimum 3.0 GPA while at Richard Stockton and a minimum grade of B in each course required for admission to the medical school; no grade below a B is accepted for required courses and classes cannot be repeated to earn a higher grade

MCAT REQUIRED

Yes, no minimum score

FINANCIAL AID

No special financial aid for students in the program

COST

	Resident Tuition and Fees ($)	Non Resident Tuition and Fees ($)
Undergraduate	12,322	18,715
Medical school	38,550	38,550

COLLEGE
Rutgers–Newark College of Arts and Sciences

MEDICAL SCHOOL
New Jersey Medical School

ADDRESS
Office of Admissions-BA/MD Program
Rutgers University
249 University Avenue, Room 100
Newark, New Jersey 07102-1808
973-353-5205
www.ncas.rutgers.edu/office-dean-student-affairs
/bamd-program-umdnj-nwk-applying

NAME OF PROGRAM
BA/MD Program

LENGTH OF PROGRAM
7 years

APPLICATION DEADLINE
November 1

INFORMATION ABOUT THE PROGRAM
This is one of eight programs associated with New Jersey Medical
School. Note that all admissions documents must be postmarked
by November 1 or they will not be considered. All documents must
be sent from high school guidance office of student in one packet.
Must be enrolled as a high school senior at time of application. In
addition to the application to the college, students must also complete a Rutgers University Self Reported Academic Record and
a BA/MD portfolio. Interviews are first conducted by Rutgers,
and if the student is recommended to the medical school, then the
medical school may also schedule an interview.

TRANSFER STUDENTS CONSIDERED
No

CITIZENSHIP REQUIREMENTS
U.S. citizen or permanent resident visa

MINIMUM REQUIRED FACTORS IN SELECTION

CLASSES

No specific requirement

GPA

Top ten percent of high school class

SAT

1,400 critical reading and math

ACT

32; writing section required

2011–2012 ACCEPTANCES

	In State	Out of State	Total
Applicants			400
Interviewed			80
New students			20

Note: these numbers reflect applications and admissions for all eight programs associated with New Jersey Medical School.

FACTORS REQUIRED TO CONTINUE IN PROGRAM

None listed

MCAT REQUIRED

Yes; no minimum score required

FINANCIAL AID

No special financial aid for students in the program

COST

	Resident Tuition and Fees ($)	Non Resident Tuition and Fees ($)
Undergraduate	13,073	26,393
Medical school	38,550	38,550

COLLEGE

Stevens Institute of Technology

MEDICAL SCHOOL

New Jersey Medical School

ADDRESS

Director of Honors Admissions Programs
Stevens Institute of Technology
Castle Point on Hudson
Hoboken, New Jersey 07030-5991
201-216-5163
www.stevens.edu/sit/admissions/academics/preprofessional.cfm

NAME OF PROGRAM

Accelerated Combined Degree Programs

LENGTH OF PROGRAM

7 years

APPLICATION DEADLINE

January 1

INFORMATION ABOUT THE PROGRAM

This is one of eight programs associated with New Jersey Medical School. Students in the program take a specific program of courses at Stevens that includes course overloads. Students major in chemical biology. An interview at Stevens is required, and you may also be asked to interview with the medical school.

TRANSFER STUDENTS CONSIDERED

No

CITIZENSHIP REQUIREMENTS

U.S. citizen or permanent resident visa

MINIMUM REQUIRED FACTORS IN SELECTION

CLASSES

Four years of English; four years of math through at least pre-calculus; one year each of biology, chemistry, and physics; AP biology and AP chemistry are recommended if available

GPA

Top ten percent of high school class

SAT

1,400 critical reading and math in one sitting; subject test in math, level 1 or 2, and chemistry or biology also required

ACT

No specific requirement

2011–2012 ACCEPTANCES

	In State	Out of State	Total
Applicants			400
Interviewed			80
New students			20

Note: these numbers reflect applications and admissions for all eight programs associated with New Jersey Medical School.

FACTORS REQUIRED TO CONTINUE IN PROGRAM

None listed

MCAT REQUIRED

Yes; no minimum required

FINANCIAL AID

No special financial aid for students in the program

COST

	Resident Tuition and Fees ($)	Non Resident Tuition and Fees ($)
Undergraduate	41,670	41,670
Medical school	38,550	38,550

COLLEGE
University of New Mexico

MEDICAL SCHOOL
University of New Mexico School of Medicine

ADDRESS
SOM Director, Combined BA/MD Program
1 University of New Mexico, MSC 09 5065
Albuquerque, New Mexico 87131-0001
505-925-4500
http://hsc.unm.edu/som/combinedbamd/

NAME OF PROGRAM
Combined BA/MD Program

LENGTH OF PROGRAM
8 years

APPLICATION DEADLINE
November 15

INFORMATION ABOUT THE PROGRAM
This program is open to New Mexico residents who are willing to
make a commitment to stay and practice medicine in New Mexico
after medical school. Factors considered for admission include
academic excellence, community involvement and volunteer service, a commitment to practice in New Mexico, honors and awards,
extracurricular activities, letters of recommendation, personal
statement, and medically related experience where available. All
students meeting the minimum test scores will be interviewed for
the program.

Students in the program are not allowed to apply to any other
medical school.

For a student from New Mexico who wishes to stay in the state,
this is a great option with no cost for the undergraduate years.

TRANSFER STUDENTS CONSIDERED
No

CITIZENSHIP REQUIREMENTS
New Mexico residents who are current New Mexico high school
seniors and high school seniors outside of New Mexico who are enrolled members of the Navajo Tribe and live in the Navajo Nation.

MINIMUM REQUIRED FACTORS IN SELECTION

CLASSES

No specific requirement

GPA

No specific requirement

SAT

Math 510; verbal 450; composite score of 900 critical reading and math

ACT

Math 22; reading 18; science 19; English 19

2010–2011 ACCEPTANCES

	In State	Out of State	Total
Applicants	209		209
Interviewed	182		182
New students	28		28

FACTORS REQUIRED TO CONTINUE IN PROGRAM

None listed

MCAT REQUIRED

Yes; students must achieve the minimum MCAT score accepted by the school of medicine, generally about a 22; part of the program is a prep class to help students prepare for the MCAT

FINANCIAL AID

All BA/MD undergraduate students are required to apply for all available scholarships. Scholarships received will be deducted from the cost of attending and a grant will be given for the difference for all undergraduates.

COST

	Resident Tuition and Fees ($)	Non Resident Tuition and Fees ($)
Undergraduate	$0	not applicable
Medical school	16,170	not applicable

COLLEGE

City College of New York (CCNY), The Sophie Davis School of Biomedical Education

MEDICAL SCHOOL

Albany Medical College

ADDRESS

Director of Admissions
Sophie Davis School of Biomedical Education at the City College of New York
Office of Admissions, Harris Hall, 160 Convent Avenue
New York, New York 10031-9101
212-650-7718
www1.ccny.cuny.edu/prospective/med/programs
/bsmdprogram.cfm

NAME OF PROGRAM

Biomedical Education Program

LENGTH OF PROGRAM

7 years

APPLICATION DEADLINE

January 8

INFORMATION ABOUT THE PROGRAM

This program is committed to increasing the number of physicians of African-American, Hispanic and other ethnic backgrounds who have been historically underrepresented in the medical profession and to serving communities that have been historically under-served by primary care physicians. Students spend the first five years at Sophie Davis of which the first three years are the undergraduate years and the last two years are the pre-clinical portion of medical school. After the two years of pre-clinical medical school, students transfer to one of six associated medical schools (Albany Medical College; New York Medical College; New York University School of Medicine; The State University of New York Health Science Center at Brooklyn; Northeast Ohio Medical University College of Medicine; The Commonwealth Medical College). Students in the program all function as a group taking the same classes.

Students in the program must sign a commitment to provide full-time medical services upon graduation, as a primary care physician in a designated physician shortage area in the State of New York.

TRANSFER STUDENTS CONSIDERED
No

CITIZENSHIP REQUIREMENTS
U.S. citizen or permanent resident visa; New York resident

MINIMUM REQUIRED FACTORS IN SELECTION

CLASSES
No specific requirement

GPA
Minimum grade average of eighty-five percent through the first three years of high school. For recent entering class, average high school GPA was ninety-five percent.

SAT
Must submit scores; for recent entering class average critical reading was 628 and math was 666.

ACT
Must submit ACT and CUNY math test; for recent entering class average was 29.

2011–2012 ACCEPTANCES

	In State	Out of State	Total
Applicants	776		776
Interviewed	254		254
New students	78		78

FACTORS REQUIRED TO CONTINUE IN PROGRAM
Grade of B or better in all biomedical subjects and a C or better in all other academic courses.

MCAT REQUIRED
No

FINANCIAL AID
No special financial aid for students in the program

COST

	Resident Tuition and Fees ($)	Non Resident Tuition and Fees ($)
Undergraduate	5,430	not applicable
Medical school	52,160	not applicable

COLLEGE
Hofstra University

MEDICAL SCHOOL
Hofstra North Shore-LIJ School of Medicine

ADDRESS
Undergraduate Admissions
Hofstra University
Hempstead, New York 11549-1000
516-463-6600
www.hofstra.edu/Admission/adm_4plus4.html

NAME OF PROGRAM
4+4 B.A.-B.S./M.D. Program

LENGTH OF PROGRAM
8 years

APPLICATION DEADLINE
November 15

INFORMATION ABOUT THE PROGRAM
Students apply to the undergraduate college, and qualified applicants will be requested to submit a supplemental application to the program. The supplemental application will be sent in January. Students may major in any subject.

TRANSFER STUDENTS CONSIDERED
No

CITIZENSHIP REQUIREMENTS
U.S. citizen or permanent resident visa

MINIMUM REQUIRED FACTORS IN SELECTION

CLASSES

Four years of math (with calculus), four years of English, and three years of science (including chemistry and physics)

GPA

Unweighted GPA of 3.7; top ten percent of high school class if the school ranks

SAT

1,350 critical reading and math

ACT

32

2010–2011 ACCEPTANCES

	In State	Out of State	Total
Applicants			
Interviewed			
New students			

No information provided

FACTORS REQUIRED TO CONTINUE IN PROGRAM

3.6 undergraduate and science GPA; no course repeated and no grade lower than a B in a science course and no grade lower than a C in a non-science course.

MCAT REQUIRED

Yes; 30, with 9 or better on each section

FINANCIAL AID

Available for undergraduate students

COST

	Resident Tuition and Fees ($)	Non Resident Tuition and Fees ($)
Undergraduate	34,900	34,900
Medical school	45,000	45,000

COLLEGE

Rensselaer Polytechnic Institute

MEDICAL SCHOOL

Albany Medical College

ADDRESS

Dean of Undergraduate Admissions
Rensselaer Polytechnic Institute
110 Eighth Street
Troy, New York 12180-3590
518-276-6216
www.rpi.edu/dept/bio/undergraduate/physician.html

NAME OF PROGRAM

Physician-Scientist Program

LENGTH OF PROGRAM

7 years

APPLICATION DEADLINE

November 1

INFORMATION ABOUT THE PROGRAM

The focus of this program is on training physicians in medical research. Students begin research activities in the spring of their junior year at Rensselaer and continue through the summer following the first year at Albany Medical College. This involves about eight months in the laboratory. Students also take a course in the principles of research.

Rensselaer identifies top students for the program and forwards those applications to Albany Medical College. Albany selects students for interviews; and interviews are conducted in January, February and March. Admissions decisions are made in April.

Motivation to study medicine and maturity are particularly important for admission to this program.

TRANSFER STUDENTS CONSIDERED

No

CITIZENSHIP REQUIREMENTS

U.S. citizen or permanent resident visa

MINIMUM REQUIRED FACTORS IN SELECTION

CLASSES

A year each of biology, chemistry, and physics; four years of math through at least pre-calculus; four years English; and two years of social studies or history.

GPA

No specific requirement

SAT

Recommend 1,400 minimum critical reading and math; one math subject test and one subject test in biology, chemistry, or physics; average SAT score 707 for critical reading, 752 for math, and 731 for writing

ACT

Accepted as alternative to SAT

2011–2012 ACCEPTANCES

	In State	Out of State	Total
Applicants	145	323	468
Interviewed	24	34	58
New students	6	8	14

FACTORS REQUIRED TO CONTINUE IN PROGRAM

None listed

MCAT REQUIRED

No

FINANCIAL AID

Available for undergraduate students

COST

	Resident Tuition and Fees ($)	Non Resident Tuition and Fees ($)
Undergraduate	44,475	44,475
Medical school	50,155	50,155

COLLEGE
Siena College

MEDICAL SCHOOL
Albany Medical College

ADDRESS
Office of Admissions
Siena College
515 Loudon Road
Loudonville, New York 12211-1462
518-783-2423
www.siena.edu/amc

NAME OF PROGRAM
Science, Humanities and Medicine Program

LENGTH OF PROGRAM
8 years

APPLICATION DEADLINE
November 15

INFORMATION ABOUT THE PROGRAM
This program places emphasis on humanities, ethics, and community service to the medically underserved. In addition to the traditional science courses, students take courses in philosophy, ethics, decision-making, social work, medical sociology, and metaphysics. In the summer after the third year of college, students engage in nonmedical work with the disadvantaged around the world. Students graduate with a biology degree and a minor in the humanities.

Following the second year of medical school, students work in rural and inner city clinics.

Beyond academics, the admissions committee focuses on leadership, communication skills, and a commitment to service. The volunteer activities should include some health-related experience.

TRANSFER STUDENTS CONSIDERED
No

CITIZENSHIP REQUIREMENTS
U.S. citizen or permanent resident visa

MINIMUM REQUIRED FACTORS IN SELECTION

CLASSES

Four years of science including biology, chemistry, and physics. Four years of math through at least pre-calculus, with calculus preferred.

GPA

Top ten percent of class

SAT

1,950 with a minimum of 1,300 in critical reading and math. Average score of 640 on SAT critical reading and 730 on SAT math section.

ACT

30

2011–2012 ACCEPTANCES

	In State	Out of State	Total
Applicants	196	155	351
Interviewed	24	22	46
New students	8	6	14

FACTORS REQUIRED TO CONTINUE IN PROGRAM

3.5 GPA

MCAT REQUIRED

No

FINANCIAL AID

Available for undergraduate students

COST

	Resident Tuition and Fees ($)	Non Resident Tuition and Fees ($)
Undergraduate	30,200	30,200
Medical school	50,155	50,155

COLLEGE
Union College

MEDICAL SCHOOL
Albany Medical College

ADDRESS
Union College
807 Union Street
Schenectady, New York 12308-3103
518-388-6112
www.union.edu/offices/LIM/

NAME OF PROGRAM
Leadership in Medicine-Health Management Program

LENGTH OF PROGRAM
8 years

APPLICATION DEADLINE
December 1

INFORMATION ABOUT THE PROGRAM

This program is unusual in that it includes a master's degree in addition to the BS and MD degrees. The first four years are spent at Union College, where students complete a biology or chemistry major as well as a second interdepartmental major in the humanities or social sciences. Ten courses in health care management are also included as part of the undergraduate education. The undergraduate program includes two summer sessions in addition to the four years at Union. A term abroad or international experience is also expected during the college years. Students are also involved in a bioethics program and a health services practicum.

A master's degree in science or an MBA is also completed during the four years at Union College. According to the program, they prepare "physicians who will be leaders capable of addressing the managerial, moral, multicultural, and international challenges facing American medicine in the twenty-first century." The focus of the program is on three areas that future leaders in medicine must be familiar with: the economic issues facing medicine, the changing face of biomedical ethics, and the need to maintain a global perspective.

Application to Union College is through the Common Application and requires a one-page addendum to apply to the program. Union identifies top students for the program and forwards those applications to Albany Medical College. Albany selects students for interviews; and interviews are conducted in January, February, and March. Admissions decisions are made in April.

Of particular importance are the personal qualities of motivation, maturity, and personal development.

TRANSFER STUDENTS CONSIDERED

No

CITIZENSHIP REQUIREMENTS

U.S. citizen or permanent resident visa

MINIMUM REQUIRED FACTORS IN SELECTION

CLASSES

Biology, chemistry, physics

GPA

Top ten percent of high school class

SAT

1,950 minimum SAT; one science and one math subject test, with minimum score of 650 on each test; average SAT scores for new students was 687 critical reading, 742 math, and 712 writing

ACT

30

2011–2012 ACCEPTANCES

	In State	Out of State	Total
Applicants	176	223	399
Interviewed	37	34	71
New students	15	6	21

FACTORS REQUIRED TO CONTINUE IN PROGRAM

3.5 GPA

MCAT REQUIRED

No

FINANCIAL AID

Union College has need-based and merit-based financial aid

COST

	Resident Tuition and Fees ($)	Non Resident Tuition and Fees ($)
Undergraduate	52,329*	52,329*
Medical school	50,155	50,155

* Includes room and board

COLLEGE

City College of New York (CCNY), The Sophie Davis School of
Biomedical Education

MEDICAL SCHOOL

New York Medical College

ADDRESS

Director of Admissions
Sophie Davis School of Biomedical Education at the City College
of New York
Office of Admissions, Harris Hall, 160 Convent Avenue
New York, New York 10031-9101
212-650-7718
www1.ccny.cuny.edu/prospective/med/programs
/bsmdprogram.cfm

NAME OF PROGRAM

Biomedical Education Program

LENGTH OF PROGRAM

7 years

APPLICATION DEADLINE

January 8

INFORMATION ABOUT THE PROGRAM

This program is committed to increasing the number of physicians
of African-American, Hispanic and other ethnic backgrounds who
have been historically underrepresented in the medical profession
and to serving communities that have been historically underserved by primary care physicians. Students spend the first five
years at Sophie Davis of which the first three years are the undergraduate years and the last two years are the pre-clinical portion of medical school. After the two years of pre-clinical medical
school, students transfer to one of six associated medical schools
(Albany Medical College; New York Medical College; New York
University School of Medicine; The State University of New York
Health Science Center at Brooklyn; Northeast Ohio Medical University College of Medicine; The Commonwealth Medical College).
Students in the program all function as a group taking the same
classes.

Students in the program must sign a commitment to provide
full-time medical services upon graduation, as a primary care
physician in a designated physician shortage area in the State of
New York.

TRANSFER STUDENTS CONSIDERED

No

CITIZENSHIP REQUIREMENTS

U.S. citizen or permanent resident visa; New York resident

MINIMUM REQUIRED FACTORS IN SELECTION

CLASSES

No specific requirement

GPA

Minimum grade average of eighty-five percent through the first three years of high school. For recent entering class, average high school GPA was ninety-five percent.

SAT

Must submit scores; for recent entering class average critical reading was 628 and math was 666.

ACT

Must submit ACT and CUNY math test; for recent entering class average was 29.

2011–2012 ACCEPTANCES

	In State	Out of State	Total
Applicants	776		776
Interviewed	254		254
New students	78		78

FACTORS REQUIRED TO CONTINUE IN PROGRAM

Grade of B or better in all biomedical subjects and a C or better in all other academic courses.

MCAT REQUIRED

No

FINANCIAL AID

No special financial aid for students in the program

COST

	Resident Tuition and Fees ($)	Non Resident Tuition and Fees ($)
Undergraduate	5,430	not applicable
Medical school	49,066	not applicable

COLLEGE

City College of New York (CCNY), The Sophie Davis School of
Biomedical Education

MEDICAL SCHOOL

New York University School of Medicine

ADDRESS

Director of Admissions
Sophie Davis School of Biomedical Education at the City College
of New York
Office of Admissions, Harris Hall, 160 Convent Avenue
New York, New York 10031-9101
212-650-7718
www1.ccny.cuny.edu/prospective/med/programs
/bsmdprogram.cfm

NAME OF PROGRAM

Biomedical Education Program

LENGTH OF PROGRAM

7 years

APPLICATION DEADLINE

January 8

INFORMATION ABOUT THE PROGRAM

This program is committed to increasing the number of physicians
of African-American, Hispanic and other ethnic backgrounds who
have been historically underrepresented in the medical profession
and to serving communities that have been historically underserved by primary care physicians. Students spend the first five
years at Sophie Davis of which the first three years are the undergraduate years and the last two years are the pre-clinical portion of medical school. After the two years of pre-clinical medical
school, students transfer to one of six associated medical schools
(Albany Medical College; New York Medical College; New York
University School of Medicine; The State University of New York
Health Science Center at Brooklyn; Northeast Ohio Medical University College of Medicine; The Commonwealth Medical College).
Students in the program all function as a group taking the same
classes.

Students in the program must sign a commitment to provide
full-time medical services upon graduation, as a primary care
physician in a designated physician shortage area in the State of
New York.

TRANSFER STUDENTS CONSIDERED

No

CITIZENSHIP REQUIREMENTS

U.S. citizen or permanent resident visa; New York resident

MINIMUM REQUIRED FACTORS IN SELECTION

CLASSES

No specific requirement

GPA

Minimum grade average of eighty-five percent through the first three years of high school. For recent entering class, average high school GPA was ninety-five percent.

SAT

Must submit scores; for recent entering class average critical reading was 628 and math was 666.

ACT

Must submit ACT and CUNY math test; for recent entering class average was 29.

2011–2012 ACCEPTANCES

	In State	Out of State	Total
Applicants	776		776
Interviewed	254		254
New students	78		78

FACTORS REQUIRED TO CONTINUE IN PROGRAM

Grade of B or better in all biomedical subjects and a C or better in all other academic courses

MCAT REQUIRED

No

FINANCIAL AID

No special financial aid for students in the program

COST

	Resident Tuition and Fees ($)	Non Resident Tuition and Fees ($)
Undergraduate	5,430	not applicable
Medical school	49,560	not applicable

COLLEGE

Brooklyn College

MEDICAL SCHOOL

The State University of New York (SUNY) Health Science
Center at Brooklyn

ADDRESS

Director, B.A.-M.D. Program
22231 Boylan Hall, Brooklyn College
2900 Bedford Avenue
Brooklyn, New York 11210-2889
718-951-4706
http://bamd.brooklyn.cuny.edu/bamdmain.html

NAME OF PROGRAM

B.A.-M.D. Program

LENGTH OF PROGRAM

8 years

APPLICATION DEADLINE

December 31

INFORMATION ABOUT THE PROGRAM

Students in the program are encouraged to major in a non-science
field. If they do major in a science-related field, they must have a
non-science minor. Students must complete a clinical internship of
320 hours during any summer except the summer following senior
year; 60 hours of non-clinical community service is required each
semester after freshman year.

TRANSFER STUDENTS CONSIDERED

No

CITIZENSHIP REQUIREMENTS

U.S. citizen or permanent resident visa; must be a resident of New
York, New Jersey, or Connecticut, with preference given to New
York State residents

MINIMUM REQUIRED FACTORS IN SELECTION

CLASSES

No specific requirement

GPA

Academic average of 90

SAT

1,200 critical reading and math; typical scores of accepted students are between 1,300 and 1,450 on critical reading and math.

ACT

No specific requirement

2011–2012 ACCEPTANCES

	In State	Out of State	Total
Applicants	305	5	310
Interviewed	88	2	90
New students	15	0	15

FACTORS REQUIRED TO CONTINUE IN PROGRAM

3.5 overall and science GPA each semester after freshman year

MCAT REQUIRED

Yes; minimum of 10 on each section of the MCAT

FINANCIAL AID

All students admitted to the program are provided a $4,000 scholarship.

COST

	Resident Tuition and Fees ($)	Non Resident Tuition and Fees ($)
Undergraduate	5,430	14,550
Medical school	29,530	54,650

COLLEGE

City College of New York (CCNY), The Sophie Davis School of Biomedical Education

MEDICAL SCHOOL

The State University of New York (SUNY) Health Science Center at Brooklyn

ADDRESS

Director of Admissions
Sophie Davis School of Biomedical Education at the City College of New York
Office of Admissions, Harris Hall, 160 Convent Avenue
New York, New York 10031-9101
212-650-7718
www1.ccny.cuny.edu/prospective/med/programs
/bsmdprogram.cfm

NAME OF PROGRAM

Biomedical Education Program

LENGTH OF PROGRAM

7 years

APPLICATION DEADLINE

January 8

INFORMATION ABOUT THE PROGRAM

This program is committed to increasing the number of physicians of African-American, Hispanic and other ethnic backgrounds who have been historically underrepresented in the medical profession and to serving communities that have been historically under-served by primary care physicians. Students spend the first five years at Sophie Davis of which the first three years are the undergraduate years and the last two years are the pre-clinical portion of medical school. After the two years of pre-clinical medical school, students transfer to one of six associated medical schools (Albany Medical College; New York Medical College; New York University School of Medicine; The State University of New York Health Science Center at Brooklyn; Northeast Ohio Medical University College of Medicine; The Commonwealth Medical College). Students in the program all function as a group taking the same classes.

Students in the program must sign a commitment to provide full-time medical services upon graduation, as a primary care physician in a designated physician shortage area in the State of New York.

TRANSFER STUDENTS CONSIDERED

No

CITIZENSHIP REQUIREMENTS

U.S. citizen or permanent resident visa; New York resident

MINIMUM REQUIRED FACTORS IN SELECTION

CLASSES

No specific requirement

GPA

Minimum grade average of eighty-five percent through the first three years of high school. For recent entering class, average high school GPA was ninety-five percent.

SAT

Must submit scores; for recent entering class average critical reading was 628 and math was 666.

ACT

Must submit ACT and CUNY math test; for recent entering class average was 29.

2011–2012 ACCEPTANCES

	In State	Out of State	Total
Applicants	776		776
Interviewed	254		254
New students	78		78

FACTORS REQUIRED TO CONTINUE IN PROGRAM

Grade of B or better in all biomedical subjects and a C or better in all other academic courses.

MCAT REQUIRED

No

FINANCIAL AID

No special financial aid for students in the program

COST

	Resident Tuition and Fees ($)	Non Resident Tuition and Fees ($)
Undergraduate	5,430	not applicable
Medical school	29,967	not applicable

COLLEGE
Stony Brook University

MEDICAL SCHOOL
Stony Brook University School of Medicine

ADDRESS
Undergraduate Admissions, Honors Programs
118 Administration Building
Stony Brook University
Stony Brook, New York 11794-1901
631-632-6868
www.stonybrook.edu/ugadmissions/newhonors
/scholarsmed.shtml

NAME OF PROGRAM
Scholars for Medicine Program

LENGTH OF PROGRAM
8 years

APPLICATION DEADLINE
January 15

INFORMATION ABOUT THE PROGRAM
Students may enter this program from one of three tracks including the Honors College, the Women in Science and Engineering (WISE) or the Engineering Program. Students may only apply to one of these programs. No specific majors are required. The program provides a series of seminars related to health-related fields and students may also engage in research.

TRANSFER STUDENTS CONSIDERED
No

CITIZENSHIP REQUIREMENTS
U.S. citizen or permanent resident visa

MINIMUM REQUIRED FACTORS IN SELECTION

CLASSES

No specific requirement

GPA

Ninety-five percent or 3.8 unweighted

SAT

1,350 critical reading and math

ACT

SAT required

2011–2012 ACCEPTANCES

	In State	Out of State	Total
Applicants	527	279	806
Interviewed	20	2	22
New students	4	1	5

FACTORS REQUIRED TO CONTINUE IN PROGRAM

3.4 cumulative GPA and 3.2 science GPA; students in the College of Engineering need a minimum cumulative and science GPA of 3.2.

MCAT REQUIRED

Yes, must score at or above the national average for that test year, with no less than an 8 on any section

FINANCIAL AID

No special financial aid for students in the program

COST

	Resident Tuition and Fees ($)	Non Resident Tuition and Fees ($)
Undergraduate	7,560	18,180
Medical school	32,210	57,330

COLLEGE
Clarkson University

MEDICAL SCHOOL
SUNY Upstate Medical University

ADDRESS
Pre-Health Sciences Advisor
Room 210 Science Center
PO Box 5805
Potsdam, New York 13699-5805
315-268-2391
www.clarkson.edu/admission/upstate_medical/

NAME OF PROGRAM
Early Admission Program

LENGTH OF PROGRAM
8 years

APPLICATION DEADLINE
February 1

INFORMATION ABOUT THE PROGRAM
Preference is given to students from an underrepresented minority. Student need to provide a recommendation letter from someone who can describe the student's potential for a career in medicine.

TRANSFER STUDENTS CONSIDERED
No

CITIZENSHIP REQUIREMENTS
U.S. citizen or permanent resident visa; resident of a rural New York community

MINIMUM REQUIRED FACTORS IN SELECTION

CLASSES

No specific requirement

GPA

Ninety percent average

SAT

1,250 critical reading and math

ACT

28

2009–2010 ACCEPTANCES

	In State	Out of State	Total
Applicants	25		25
Interviewed	5		5
New students	0		0

FACTORS REQUIRED TO CONTINUE IN PROGRAM

3.5 overall and science GPA

MCAT REQUIRED

Yes; minimum score of 30

FINANCIAL AID

No special financial aid for students in the program

COST

	Resident Tuition and Fees ($)	Non Resident Tuition and Fees ($)
Undergraduate	38,610	not applicable
Medical school	29,530	not applicable

COLLEGE
Hobart and William Smith Colleges

MEDICAL SCHOOL
SUNY Upstate Medical University

ADDRESS
Pre-Health Advisor
Elizabeth Blackwell Medical Scholars Program
Hobart and William Smith Colleges
Office of Admissions, 629 South Main Street
Geneva, New York 14456-3165
800-852-2256
www.hws.edu/admissions/pdf/blackwell_scholars.pdf

NAME OF PROGRAM
Elizabeth Blackwell Medical Scholars Program

LENGTH OF PROGRAM
8 years

APPLICATION DEADLINE
January 1

INFORMATION ABOUT THE PROGRAM
To qualify for the program students must meet at least one of the following criteria: be from a rural background; be from an underrepresented minority; be the first generation to attend college. During the undergraduate years, students must complete an internship/shadowing program at related hospitals and complete enrichment opportunities offered by the medical school.

TRANSFER STUDENTS CONSIDERED
No

CITIZENSHIP REQUIREMENTS
U.S. citizen or permanent resident visa

MINIMUM REQUIRED FACTORS IN SELECTION

CLASSES

No specific requirement

GPA

3.7 unweighted or 90 on 100 scale

SAT

1,250 critical reading and math

ACT

28

2011–2012 ACCEPTANCES

	In State	Out of State	Total
Applicants	35	8	43
Interviewed	5	1	6
New students	2	0	2

FACTORS REQUIRED TO CONTINUE IN PROGRAM

3.5 GPA in sciences courses and a 3.0 GPA each semester to maintain scholarship eligibility.

MCAT REQUIRED

Yes; minimum score of 30

FINANCIAL AID

Students accepted into the program receive a full tuition scholarship for all four years of undergraduate study.

COST

	Resident Tuition and Fees ($)	Non Resident Tuition and Fees ($)
Undergraduate	12,215	not applicable
Medical school	29,530	not applicable

COLLEGE

St. Bonaventure University

MEDICAL SCHOOL

SUNY Upstate Medical University

ADDRESS

Director Franciscan Health Care Professionals Program
Biology Department
De La Roche Hall, Room 219
St. Bonaventure University
3261 West State Road
St. Bonaventure, New York 14778-9800
716-375-2656
www.sbu.edu/artsandsciences.aspx?id=20630

NAME OF PROGRAM

Dual Admission Program

LENGTH OF PROGRAM

8 years

APPLICATION DEADLINE

December 15

INFORMATION ABOUT THE PROGRAM

Preference is given to applicants from rural areas and those with a
strong desire to practice in rural and underserved areas. Students
being considered with be invited for an interview at St. Bonaventure in January or February and then invited for an interview at
the medical school in March. A personal statement essay detailing
your interest in the medical field and your interest in St. Bonaventure and Upstate Medical Center is required. This may be one or
two essays. A résumé of all of your extracurricular activities is
also required as are two letters of recommendation including at
least one from a science teacher.

TRANSFER STUDENTS CONSIDERED

No

CITIZENSHIP REQUIREMENTS

U.S. citizen or permanent resident visa; New York residents only

MINIMUM REQUIRED FACTORS IN SELECTION

CLASSES

No specific requirement

GPA

90 on 100 scale

SAT

1,300 critical reading and math

ACT

29

2011–2012 ACCEPTANCES

	In State	Out of State	Total
Applicants			
Interviewed	3		3
New students	2		2

FACTORS REQUIRED TO CONTINUE IN PROGRAM

3.5 minimum GPA overall and in science courses; no grade lower than B–

MCAT REQUIRED

Yes; minimum score of 30

FINANCIAL AID

No special financial aid for students in the program.

COST

	Resident Tuition and Fees ($)	Non Resident Tuition and Fees ($)
Undergraduate	28,727	not applicable
Medical school	29,530	not applicable

COLLEGE
St. Lawrence University

MEDICAL SCHOOL
SUNY Upstate Medical University

ADDRESS
Director of Admissions
St. Lawrence University
23 Romoda Drive
Canton, New York 13617-1423
800-285-1856
www.stlawu.edu/admis/rmed.html

NAME OF PROGRAM
Rural Medicine Program

LENGTH OF PROGRAM
8 years

APPLICATION DEADLINE
December 1

INFORMATION ABOUT THE PROGRAM
Strong preference is given to applicants from a rural setting who are also first generation college students or from a disadvantaged economic background. Strong preference is also given to those students who have a desire to return to practice medicine in an underserved rural area. Volunteer service and doctor shadowing during the undergraduate years are also required.

Students complete an application to the college and a separate application to the program.

TRANSFER STUDENTS CONSIDERED
No

CITIZENSHIP REQUIREMENTS
U.S. citizen or permanent resident visa; preference given to residents of rural New York

MINIMUM REQUIRED FACTORS IN SELECTION

CLASSES
No specific requirement

GPA
Ninety percent average

SAT
1,250 critical reading and math

ACT
27

2010–2011 ACCEPTANCES

	In State	Out of State	Total
Applicants	4		4
Interviewed	2		2
New students	1		1

FACTORS REQUIRED TO CONTINUE IN PROGRAM
Overall and science GPA of 3.5

MCAT REQUIRED
Yes, minimum score of 30

FINANCIAL AID
No special financial aid for students in the program.

COST

	Resident Tuition and Fees ($)	Non Resident Tuition and Fees ($)
Undergraduate	44,075	44,075
Medical school	29,530	54,650

COLLEGE
SUNY Cobleskill

MEDICAL SCHOOL
SUNY Upstate Medical University

ADDRESS
SUNY Cobleskill
State Route 7
Cobleskill, New York 12043-1704
518-255-5011
www.cobleskill.edu/academics/student-success-center
/med-school.asp

NAME OF PROGRAM
Medical School Early Assurance Program

LENGTH OF PROGRAM
8 years

APPLICATION DEADLINE
January 5

INFORMATION ABOUT THE PROGRAM
Preference given to students who come from a rural area of New York State and come from a disadvantaged background. Students accepted into the program will participate in the Rural Medical Scholars Program.

Students in the program will spend two years at SUNY Cobleskill, two years at either Siena College or Cornell University College of Agricultural and Life Sciences, and the remaining time at SUNY Upstate Medical University.

TRANSFER STUDENTS CONSIDERED
No

CITIZENSHIP REQUIREMENTS
U.S. citizen or permanent resident visa; New York State residents

MINIMUM REQUIRED FACTORS IN SELECTION

CLASSES

Three years math and science

GPA

90 out of 100

SAT

1,300 critical reading and math

ACT

29

2010–2011 ACCEPTANCES

	In State	Out of State	Total
Applicants			
Interviewed			
New students			

No information provided

FACTORS REQUIRED TO CONTINUE IN PROGRAM

Over all and science GPA of 3.5

MCAT REQUIRED

Yes; minimum score of 30

FINANCIAL AID

No special financial aid for students in the program

COST

	Resident Tuition and Fees ($)	Non Resident Tuition and Fees ($)
Undergraduate	6,819 Cobleskill	not applicable
Medical school	29,530	not applicable

COLLEGE
SUNY College of Environmental Science and Forestry

MEDICAL SCHOOL
SUNY Upstate Medical University

ADDRESS
SUNY-ESF
1 Forestry Drive
Syracuse, New York 13210-2712
315-470-6600
www.esf.edu/prehealth/umu.htm

NAME OF PROGRAM
Joint BS/MD Program

LENGTH OF PROGRAM
8 years

APPLICATION DEADLINE
February 1

INFORMATION ABOUT THE PROGRAM
This program addresses the shortage of physicians in rural New York. The program also is trying to provide a more diverse student population for entry into medical school. Students in the program will participate in the Rural Medical Scholars Program. Students may major in any program.

TRANSFER STUDENTS CONSIDERED
No

CITIZENSHIP REQUIREMENTS
U.S. citizen or permanent resident visa; New York state residency. Preference given to students from a rural county.

MINIMUM REQUIRED FACTORS IN SELECTION

CLASSES

No specific requirements

GPA

90 out of 100 GPA

SAT

1,250 critical reading and math

ACT

28

2010–2011 ACCEPTANCES

	In State	Out of State	Total
Applicants			
Interviewed			
New students			

No information provided

FACTORS REQUIRED TO CONTINUE IN PROGRAM

Overall and science GPA of 3.5

MCAT REQUIRED

Yes; minimum score of 30

FINANCIAL AID

No special financial aid for students in the program

COST

	Resident Tuition and Fees ($)	Non Resident Tuition and Fees ($)
Undergraduate	6,492	not applicable
Medical school	29,530	not applicable

COLLEGE

SUNY Geneseo

MEDICAL SCHOOL

SUNY Upstate Medical University

ADDRESS

Director of Admissions
SUNY Geneseo
1 College Circle
Geneseo, New York 14454-1401
585-245-5000
www.geneseo.edu/admissions/bsmd-suny-upstate

NAME OF PROGRAM

BS/MD Early Admittance Program

LENGTH OF PROGRAM

8 years

APPLICATION DEADLINE

January 1

INFORMATION ABOUT THE PROGRAM

Preference given to students who are from a rural community in
New York State and who come from a disadvantaged background.
However, students from more urban backgrounds are also considered. The program is geared to students who wish to practice
family medicine in rural communities after graduation. Students
applying to the program should select biology as your major and
notify the admissions office of your interest in the program. There
is also a required essay detailing your interest and experience in
the health field and your interest in the program through Geneseo. This essay may be emailed to the admissions office.

There are various experiences provided to help support students before attending medical school.

TRANSFER STUDENTS CONSIDERED

No

CITIZENSHIP REQUIREMENTS

U.S. citizen or permanent resident visa; New York resident

MINIMUM REQUIRED FACTORS IN SELECTION

CLASSES

No specific requirement

GPA

Ninety percent average

SAT

1,250 critical reading and math

ACT

28

2011–2012 ACCEPTANCES

	In State	Out of State	Total
Applicants	55		55
Interviewed	6		6
New students	3		3

FACTORS REQUIRED TO CONTINUE IN PROGRAM

3.5 overall and science GPA

MCAT REQUIRED

Yes; minimum score of 30

FINANCIAL AID

No special financial aid for students in the program

COST

	Resident Tuition and Fees ($)	Non Resident Tuition and Fees ($)
Undergraduate	7,095	not applicable
Medical school	29,530	not applicable

COLLEGE
SUNY Potsdam

MEDICAL SCHOOL
SUNY Upstate Medical University

ADDRESS
Director of Admissions
State University of New York at Potsdam
44 Pierrepont Avenue
Potsdam, New York 13676-2200
315-267-2000
www.upstate.edu/com/admissions/options/potsdam.php

NAME OF PROGRAM
Special Admissions Options

LENGTH OF PROGRAM
8 years

APPLICATION DEADLINE
No information provided

INFORMATION ABOUT THE PROGRAM
Preference given to students who come from a rural area of New York State and come from a disadvantaged background. Students accepted into the program will participate in the Rural Medical Scholars Program.

TRANSFER STUDENTS CONSIDERED
No

CITIZENSHIP REQUIREMENTS
U.S. citizen or permanent resident visa, New York State residents

MINIMUM REQUIRED FACTORS IN SELECTION

CLASSES
No specific requirements

GPA
90 out of 100

SAT
1,250 critical reading and math

ACT
28

2010–2011 ACCEPTANCES

	In State	Out of State	Total
Applicants			
Interviewed			
New students			

No information provided

FACTORS REQUIRED TO CONTINUE IN PROGRAM
Overall and science GPA of 3.5

MCAT REQUIRED
Yes; minimum score of 30

FINANCIAL AID
No special financial aid for students in the program

COST

	Resident Tuition and Fees ($)	Non Resident Tuition and Fees ($)
Undergraduate	6,835	not applicable
Medical school	29,530	not applicable

COLLEGE
Wilkes University

MEDICAL SCHOOL
SUNY Upstate Medical University

ADDRESS
Wilkes University
84 West South Street
Wilkes-Barre, Pennsylvanian 18766-0003
800-945-5378
www.upstate.edu/com/admissions/options/guthrie.php

NAME OF PROGRAM
Guthrie Pre-Medical Scholars Program

LENGTH OF PROGRAM
8 years

APPLICATION DEADLINE
November 15

INFORMATION ABOUT THE PROGRAM
The purpose of this program is to increase the number of physicians interested in serving in rural health care delivery systems. This program requires three interviews including one at Wilkes, one at a local clinical site, and one at the SUNY Upstate medical school.

TRANSFER STUDENTS CONSIDERED
No

CITIZENSHIP REQUIREMENTS
U.S. citizen or permanent resident visa; must reside in a rural county in the Southern Tier of New York State

MINIMUM REQUIRED FACTORS IN SELECTION

CLASSES

Four years of math, English, science, and social studies

GPA

Top ten percent of high school class

SAT

1,200 critical reading and math

ACT

27

2011–2012 ACCEPTANCES

	In State	Out of State	Total
Applicants	1		1
Interviewed	1		1
New students	1		1

FACTORS REQUIRED TO CONTINUE IN PROGRAM

3.5 overall and science GPA

MCAT REQUIRED

Yes; minimum score of 30

FINANCIAL AID

No special financial aid for students in the program

COST

	Resident Tuition and Fees ($)	Non Resident Tuition and Fees ($)
Undergraduate	29,326	not applicable
Medical school	29,530	not applicable

COLLEGE
University of Rochester

MEDICAL SCHOOL
University of Rochester School of Medicine

ADDRESS
Office of Admissions
PO Box 270251
Rochester, New York 14627-0251
585-275-3221
http://enrollment.rochester.edu/admissions/CAPs/REMS/

NAME OF PROGRAM
Rochester Early Medical Scholars (REMS)

LENGTH OF PROGRAM
8 years

APPLICATION DEADLINE
December 1

INFORMATION ABOUT THE PROGRAM
Students in the REMS program may major in any subject and are encouraged to explore all of the academic offerings of the university. The most popular majors are biology, chemistry, and health and society. Students are required to complete a social service project before enrolling in the medical school. REMS students may also apply to any of the other combined degree programs available at the University including MD/PhD, MD/MPH, MD/MBA and MD/MS programs.

The school of medicine's Double-Helix curriculum integrates the basic science and clinical science aspects of medical school across all four years of the medical school experience. This means that the medical students begin clinical clerkships in January of the first year. The medical school encourages critical thinking, problem solving, and active learning in small groups.

Summer research programs and international experiences are available for REMS undergraduates and medical students.

Advantages of the REMS program include faculty mentors; seminars; support and social events; academic freedom; problem-based learning; and funding for summer research.

TRANSFER STUDENTS CONSIDERED
No

CITIZENSHIP REQUIREMENTS
International students considered for program

MINIMUM REQUIRED FACTORS IN SELECTION

CLASSES

No specific requirement

GPA

No minimum but the strongest applicants have a 3.95 unweighted GPA with strong college prep courses and top three percent of their high school class.

SAT

No minimum but strongest applicants have at least a 1,450 SAT score on the critical reading and math and at least 700 on SAT writing. Average SAT critical reading score is 729, average SAT math score is 751, and average writing score is 756.

SAT SUBJECT TESTS

No minimum and not required. However, applicants are strongly encouraged to take a subject test in biology or chemistry and a subject test in math level 1 or math level 2. Strongest applicants score 700 or above on each of these subject tests.

ACT

No minimum but strongest applicants have at least a 34.

2011–2012 ACCEPTANCES

	In State	Out of State	Total
Applicants	135	259	394
Interviewed	12	34	46
New students	7	3	10

FACTORS REQUIRED TO CONTINUE IN PROGRAM

Students must have an overall GPA of 3.3 and a math and science GPA of 3.3 after freshman year, a 3.4 GPA overall and in math and science courses after sophomore year, and a 3.5 overall GPA and math and science GPA after junior year in college.

MCAT REQUIRED

No

FINANCIAL AID

The University of Rochester meets one hundred percent of the demonstrated need for a student's undergraduate education.

COST

	Resident Tuition and Fees ($)	Non Resident Tuition and Fees ($)
Undergraduate	43,636	43,636
Medical school	44,700	44,700

COLLEGE
East Carolina University

MEDICAL SCHOOL
East Carolina University Brody School of Medicine

ADDRESS
Office of Admissions
East Carolina University
600 Moye Boulevard
Greenville, North Carolina 27834-4300
252-328-6373
www.ecu.edu/bsomadmissions/assurance.cfm

NAME OF PROGRAM
Early Assurance Program

LENGTH OF PROGRAM
8 years

APPLICATION DEADLINE
December 1

INFORMATION ABOUT THE PROGRAM
Students must be admitted to the Honors College to be considered for the program. There are numerous group and enrichment activities for students in the program, including hands-on medical exposure, summer programs, and service learning.

TRANSFER STUDENTS CONSIDERED
No

CITIZENSHIP REQUIREMENTS
U.S. citizen or permanent resident visa; North Carolina residents only

MINIMUM REQUIRED FACTORS IN SELECTION

CLASSES

No specific requirement

GPA

3.5 unweighted or 4.0 weighted

SAT

1,200

ACT

26

2010–2011 ACCEPTANCES

	In State	Out of State	Total
Applicants	80		80
Interviewed	24		24
New students	4		4

FACTORS REQUIRED TO CONTINUE IN PROGRAM

3.5 overall and science GPA

MCAT REQUIRED

No

FINANCIAL AID

No special financial aid for students in the program

COST

	Resident Tuition and Fees ($)	Non Resident Tuition and Fees ($)
Undergraduate	5,332	not applicable
Medical school	14,695	not applicable

COLLEGE

Case Western Reserve University

MEDICAL SCHOOL

Case Western Reserve University School of Medicine

ADDRESS

Office of Undergraduate Admission
Wolstein Hall, Case Western Reserve University
10900 Euclid Avenue
Cleveland, Ohio 44106-7055
216-368-4450
http://admission.case.edu/academics/ppsp.aspx

NAME OF PROGRAM

Pre-Professional Scholars Program

LENGTH OF PROGRAM

8 years

APPLICATION DEADLINE

December 1

INFORMATION ABOUT THE PROGRAM

Students who complete the undergraduate program in less than four years may not enter the medical school early. They are required to spend any available time involved in experiences that will enhance their personal or professional development. No specific majors are required, although the most common are biology and biochemistry.

TRANSFER STUDENTS CONSIDERED

No

CITIZENSHIP REQUIREMENTS

International students considered

MINIMUM REQUIRED FACTORS IN SELECTION

CLASSES

One year each of biology, chemistry, and physics as well as four years of math

GPA

No minimum, although typical candidates are in the top ten percent of their high school class

SAT

No minimum, although typical candidates score between 2,200 and 2,300 on SAT; for the fall 2010 entering class, scores ranged from 680 to 800 on critical reading, 710 to 800 on math, and 710 to 800 on writing

ACT

No minimum, although typical candidates score between 33 and 36

2011–2012 ACCEPTANCES

	In State	Out of State	Total
Applicants	134	535	669
Interviewed	4	41	45
New students	1	1	2

FACTORS REQUIRED TO CONTINUE IN PROGRAM

B+ level of performance in college coursework

MCAT REQUIRED

No; students who choose to take it must score 33 or above; MCAT is required for some scholarship programs.

FINANCIAL AID

No special financial aid for students in the program

COST

	Resident Tuition and Fees ($)	Non Resident Tuition and Fees ($)
Undergraduate	40,120	40,120
Medical school	51,450	51,450

COLLEGE

City College of New York (CCNY), The Sophie Davis School of
Biomedical Education

MEDICAL SCHOOL

Northeast Ohio Medical University

ADDRESS

Director of Admissions
Sophie Davis School of Biomedical Education at the City College
of New York
Office of Admissions, Harris Hall, 160 Convent Avenue
New York, New York 10031-9101
212-650-7718
www1.ccny.cuny.edu/prospective/med/programs
/bsmdprogram.cfm

NAME OF PROGRAM

Biomedical Education Program

LENGTH OF PROGRAM

7 years

APPLICATION DEADLINE

January 8

INFORMATION ABOUT THE PROGRAM

This program is committed to increasing the number of physicians
of African-American, Hispanic and other ethnic backgrounds who
have been historically underrepresented in the medical profession
and to serving communities that have been historically underserved by primary care physicians. Students spend the first five
years at Sophie Davis of which the first three years are the undergraduate years and the last two years are the pre-clinical portion of medical school. After the two years of pre-clinical medical
school, students transfer to one of six associated medical schools
(Albany Medical College; New York Medical College; New York
University School of Medicine; The State University of New York
Health Science Center at Brooklyn; Northeast Ohio Medical University College of Medicine; The Commonwealth Medical College)
Students in the program all function as a group taking the same
classes.

Students in the program must sign a commitment to provide
full-time medical services upon graduation, as a primary care
physician in a designated physician shortage area in the State of
New York.

TRANSFER STUDENTS CONSIDERED

No

CITIZENSHIP REQUIREMENTS

U.S. citizen or permanent resident visa; New York resident

MINIMUM REQUIRED FACTORS IN SELECTION

CLASSES

No specific requirement

GPA

Minimum grade average of eighty-five percent through the first three years of high school. For recent entering class, average high school GPA was ninety-five percent.

SAT

Must submit scores; for recent entering class average critical reading was 628 and math was 666.

ACT

Must submit ACT and CUNY math test; for recent entering class average was 28.

2011–2012 ACCEPTANCES

	In State	Out of State	Total
Applicants	776		776
Interviewed	254		254
New students	78		78

FACTORS REQUIRED TO CONTINUE IN PROGRAM

Grade of B or better in all biomedical subjects and a C or better in all other academic courses.

MCAT REQUIRED

No

FINANCIAL AID

No special financial aid for students in the program

COST

	Resident Tuition and Fees ($)	Non Resident Tuition and Fees ($)
Undergraduate	5,430	not applicable
Medical school	34,455	not applicable

COLLEGE

Kent State University; University of Akron;
Youngstown State University

MEDICAL SCHOOL

Northeast Ohio Medical University

ADDRESS

Office of Admissions
Northeast Ohio Medical University
4209 State Route 44
PO Box 95
Rootstown, Ohio 44272-0095
330-325-6270
www.neomed.edu/admissions/medicine/bsmd

NAME OF PROGRAM

B.S./M.D. Program

LENGTH OF PROGRAM

6 or 7 years

APPLICATION DEADLINE

December 15; early action deadline October 15

INFORMATION ABOUT THE PROGRAM

Unlike most other programs, the student applies to the medical
school directly and, if chosen, is assigned a college for the first
two to three years of the program. Each college is given thirty-five
students from the program for a total class of 105. Strong preference is given to Ohio residents and in particular those students
who are interested in primary medicine in the Northeast Ohio
area. No more than ten percent of the class is from outside Ohio.
Students have the option of completing the undergraduate portion of the program in two or three years. The program will not
consider any materials or letters of recommendation beyond what
they specifically request.

TRANSFER STUDENTS CONSIDERED

No

CITIZENSHIP REQUIREMENTS

U.S. citizen or permanent resident visa; preference given to Ohio
residents

MINIMUM REQUIRED FACTORS IN SELECTION

CLASSES

Four years of math, science, English, social studies, and a foreign language are recommended.

GPA

3.5; accepted student average 3.88; 25th to 75th percentile is 3.81 to 4.00.

SAT

Accepted students average 1,371; 25th to 75th percentile is 1,308 to 1,455 on the critical reading and math sections.

ACT

27; accepted students average 31; 25th to 75th percentile is 29 to 32.

2011–2012 ACCEPTANCES

	In State	Out of State	Total
Applicants	298	197	495
Interviewed	199	21	220
New students	102	4	106

FACTORS REQUIRED TO CONTINUE IN PROGRAM

Students must have a 3.2 science and math GPA and a 3.25 overall GPA and earn at least an 8 on each section of the MCAT to advance to the medical school after two or three years. If you have a 3.5 overall and science and math GPA, you can advance with an MCAT score of 24 with one score of 7.

MCAT REQUIRED

Yes; must receive at least an 8 on each section of the test

FINANCIAL AID

There are merit-based scholarships available.

COST

	Resident Tuition and Fees ($)	Non Resident Tuition and Fees ($)
Undergraduate	varies	varies
Medical school	34,455	66,410

COLLEGE
University of Cincinnati

MEDICAL SCHOOL
University of Cincinnati College of Medicine

ADDRESS
University of Cincinnati
231 Albert Sabin Way
Cincinnati, Ohio 45267-2827
513-558-5581
http://med.uc.edu/DualAdmissions.aspx

NAME OF PROGRAM
Connections Program

LENGTH OF PROGRAM
8 years

APPLICATION DEADLINE
November 30

INFORMATION ABOUT THE PROGRAM
Students must also participate as members of the honors program
at the university. The program is not binding, and students in the
college may apply to other medical schools without penalty. There
are various enrichment opportunities available for students in the
program. Students must complete both the university undergraduate application as well as the Connection Program application.
These are separate applications.

TRANSFER STUDENTS CONSIDERED
No

CITIZENSHIP REQUIREMENTS
U.S. citizen or permanent resident visa; preference given to Ohio
residents

MINIMUM REQUIRED FACTORS IN SELECTION

CLASSES

No specific requirement

GPA

No specific requirement; average GPA of admitted students is 4.33.

SAT

1,300 critical reading and math; average SAT of students admitted to the program is 1,423.

ACT

29; average ACT of students admitted to the program is 33.

2011–2012 ACCEPTANCES

	In State	Out of State	Total
Applicants			181
Interviewed			32
New students	7	4	11

FACTORS REQUIRED TO CONTINUE IN PROGRAM

3.45 science GPA and 3.4 overall GPA; graduation from the University Honors Program

MCAT REQUIRED

Yes; minimum score of 30 with no less than a 9 in any section

FINANCIAL AID

No special financial aid for students in the program

COST

	Resident Tuition and Fees ($)	Non Resident Tuition and Fees ($)
Undergraduate	10,784	25,816
Medical school	30,597	48,327

COLLEGE
University of Toledo

MEDICAL SCHOOL
University of Toledo College of Medicine

ADDRESS
University of Toledo
Department of Bioengineering
5051 Nitschke Hall MS 303
2801 West Bancroft Street
Toledo, OH 43606-3390
419-530-8078
www.bioe.eng.utoledo.edu/undergraduate/programs/bsmd.html

Baccalaureate/MD Program Advisor
University of Toledo
2801 West Bancroft Street
Toledo, Ohio 43606-3390
419-530-2102
www.utoledo.edu/offices/studentservices/preprofessional
/Baccalaureate_MD_Program.html

NAME OF PROGRAM
Baccalaureate/MD Program and BS/MD Program

LENGTH OF PROGRAM
7, 8, or 9 years

APPLICATION DEADLINE
November 30 for the BS/MD Program; December 1 for the Bac/
MD program

INFORMATION ABOUT THE PROGRAM
This is actually two different programs with similar admission
requirements. The Baccalaureate/MD program is for students in
The College of Natural Science and Mathematics, The College of
Literature, Languages, and Social Sciences and the College of Vi-
sual and Performing Arts. This program lasts seven or eight years
depending on advanced placement credits that the student starts
with and the major the student chooses. There are typically about
five seats available with this program.

The BS/MD program is through the department of bioengineering. This program lasts eight or nine years. There are three
to five semesters in co-op programs in biomedical engineering po-
sitions. There are typically about ten seats available through this
program. Students may apply to only one of the programs, not
both.

Students in each of the programs have several curriculum enhancements through the program, including medical student mentors, clinical encounters, and enhanced course work in topics related to medicine.

In addition to the application form for the University, there is a separate application form for each program.

TRANSFER STUDENTS CONSIDERED

No

CITIZENSHIP REQUIREMENTS

U.S. citizen or permanent resident visa; preference given to Ohio residents

MINIMUM REQUIRED FACTORS IN SELECTION

CLASSES

No specific requirement

GPA

3.8 unweighted; average weighted GPA for BS/MD Program was 4.2.

SAT

1,300 critical reading and math; average SAT score for BS/MD Program was 1,397.

ACT

29; average ACT score for BS/MD Program was 31.

2010–2011 ACCEPTANCES

	In State	Out of State	Total
Applicants	37 BS; ? Bacc		
Interviewed	14 BS; ? Bacc		
New students	10 BS; ? Bacc		

Note: the Department of Bioengineering provided numbers for the BS/MD program; the Baccalaureate/MD program did not provide numbers before press time.

FACTORS REQUIRED TO CONTINUE IN PROGRAM

3.5 GPA and agreement not to seek admission at another medical school

MCAT REQUIRED

No; MCAT scores required for scholarship consideration

FINANCIAL AID

No special financial aid for students in the program

COST

	Resident Tuition and Fees ($)	Non Resident Tuition and Fees ($)
Undergraduate	7,864	16,984
Medical school	30,659	60,863

COLLEGE
University of Oklahoma

MEDICAL SCHOOL
University of Oklahoma College of Medicine

ADDRESS
Program Director
Joe C. and Carol Kerr McClendon Honors College
David L. Boren Hall
1300 Asp Avenue
Norman, Oklahoma 73019-6061
405-325-5291
www.ou.edu/honors/MedicalHumanities/

NAME OF PROGRAM
Medical Humanities Scholars Program

LENGTH OF PROGRAM
7 or 8 years

APPLICATION DEADLINE
December 1

INFORMATION ABOUT THE PROGRAM
Students applying to the program must submit three separate applications. The regular application and the application to the Honors College are available online and are due by December 1. The Medical Humanities Scholars Program application is due by January 8. This application is available online, but four copies must be submitted through regular mail.

Students may major in any subject but will self-design a minor in medical humanities. During the undergraduate years students participate in mini internships with both private and academic physicians. Students are encouraged to take a full four years for the undergraduate portion of the program but may petition for approval to obtain their undergraduate degree after three years.

TRANSFER STUDENTS CONSIDERED
No

CITIZENSHIP REQUIREMENTS
U.S. citizen or permanent resident visa; must graduate from a U.S. high school

MINIMUM REQUIRED FACTORS IN SELECTION

No specific requirement

2010–2011 ACCEPTANCES

	In State	Out of State	Total
Applicants			
Interviewed			
New students			

No information provided

FACTORS REQUIRED TO CONTINUE IN PROGRAM

Student must have a GPA and MCAT score equal to or higher than the average GPA and MCAT scores of the previous year's entering class.

MCAT REQUIRED

Yes

FINANCIAL AID

No special financial aid for students in the program

COST

	Resident Tuition and Fees ($)	Non Resident Tuition and Fees ($)
Undergraduate	8,705.50	20,342.50
Medical school	22,502.50	48,972.50

COLLEGE

City College of New York (CCNY), The Sophie Davis School of
Biomedical Education

MEDICAL SCHOOL

The Commonwealth Medical College

ADDRESS

Director of Admissions
Sophie Davis School of Biomedical Education at the City College
of New York
Office of Admissions, Harris Hall, 160 Convent Avenue
New York, New York 10031-9101
212-650-7718
www1.ccny.cuny.edu/prospective/med/programs
/bsmdprogram.cfm

NAME OF PROGRAM

Biomedical Education Program

LENGTH OF PROGRAM

7 years

APPLICATION DEADLINE

January 8

INFORMATION ABOUT THE PROGRAM

This program is committed to increasing the number of physicians
of African-American, Hispanic and other ethnic backgrounds who
have been historically underrepresented in the medical profession
and to serving communities that have been historically underserved by primary care physicians. Students spend the first five
years at Sophie Davis of which the first three years are the undergraduate years and the last two years are the pre-clinical portion of medical school. After the two years of pre-clinical medical
school, students transfer to one of six associated medical schools
(Albany Medical College; New York Medical College; New York
University School of Medicine; The State University of New York
Health Science Center at Brooklyn; Northeast Ohio Medical University College of Medicine; The Commonwealth Medical College).
Students in the program all function as a group taking the same
classes.

Students in the program must sign a commitment to provide
full-time medical services upon graduation, as a primary care
physician in a designated physician shortage area in the State of
New York.

TRANSFER STUDENTS CONSIDERED

No

CITIZENSHIP REQUIREMENTS

U.S. citizen or permanent resident visa; New York resident

MINIMUM REQUIRED FACTORS IN SELECTION

CLASSES

No specific requirement

GPA

Minimum grade average of eighty-five percent through the first three years of high school. For recent entering class, average high school GPA was ninety-five percent.

SAT

Must submit scores; for recent entering class average critical reading was 628 and math was 666.

ACT

Must submit ACT and CUNY math test; for recent entering class average was 29.

2011–2012 ACCEPTANCES

	In State	Out of State	Total
Applicants	776		776
Interviewed	254		254
New students	78		78

FACTORS REQUIRED TO CONTINUE IN PROGRAM

Grade of B or better in all biomedical subjects and a C or better in all other academic courses.

MCAT REQUIRED

No

FINANCIAL AID

No special financial aid for students in the program

COST

	Resident Tuition and Fees ($)	Non Resident Tuition and Fees ($)
Undergraduate	5,430	not applicable
Medical school	53,670	not applicable

COLLEGE
University of the Sciences in Philadelphia

MEDICAL SCHOOL
The Commonwealth Medical College

ADDRESS
University of the Sciences in Philadelphia
600 South 43rd Street
Philadelphia, Pennsylvania 19104-4418
215-596-8800
www.usciences.edu/academics/programs/premed/DualDegree
/TCMC.aspx

NAME OF PROGRAM
Dual Degree Program

LENGTH OF PROGRAM
8 years

APPLICATION DEADLINE
No information provided

INFORMATION ABOUT THE PROGRAM
Students will complete any bachelor of science major. Pennsylvania residents with a history of community service are the most competitive candidates.

TRANSFER STUDENTS CONSIDERED
No

CITIZENSHIP REQUIREMENTS
U.S. citizen or permanent resident visa

MINIMUM REQUIRED FACTORS IN SELECTION

CLASSES

No specific requirements

GPA

3.40 unweighted; rank in the top twenty percent of your class

SAT

1,200 critical reading and math

ACT

25

2010–2011 ACCEPTANCES

	In State	Out of State	Total
Applicants			
Interviewed			
New students			

No information provided

FACTORS REQUIRED TO CONTINUE IN PROGRAM

No information provided

MCAT REQUIRED

No information provided

FINANCIAL AID

No special financial aid for students in the program

COST

	Resident Tuition and Fees ($)	Non Resident Tuition and Fees ($)
Undergraduate	33,406	33,406
Medical school	48,419	53,670

COLLEGE
Drexel University

MEDICAL SCHOOL
Drexel University College of Medicine

ADDRESS
Drexel University Undergraduate Admissions
PO Box 34789
Philadelphia, Pennsylvania 19101-4789
215-895-2000
www.drexel.edu/undergrad/apply/freshmen-instructions
/accelerated/

NAME OF PROGRAM
BA/BS/MD

LENGTH OF PROGRAM
7 or 8 years

APPLICATION DEADLINE
November 15

INFORMATION ABOUT THE PROGRAM
Students majoring in the biological sciences, chemistry, psychology or the bachelor of science in engineering can apply to the seven-year program. There is also an eight-year option for students majoring in biomedical engineering or general engineering. Students must submit an application to the undergraduate college as well as a College of Medicine supplemental application. Two letters of recommendation are required; one must be from a high school counselor and the other from a science teacher.

TRANSFER STUDENTS CONSIDERED
No

CITIZENSHIP REQUIREMENTS
U.S. citizen or permanent resident visa; must graduate from a U.S. high school

MINIMUM REQUIRED FACTORS IN SELECTION

CLASSES

Four years of math, English, and science, including one year each of biology, chemistry, and physics

GPA

Graduate from U.S. high school in top ten percent of class with 3.5 unweighted GPA; average high school GPA for a recent class was 3.9

SAT

1,360 critical reading and math; average SAT score for a recent class was 1,495; SAT subject tests recommended

ACT

31; average ACT score for a recent class was 34

2011–2012 ACCEPTANCES

	In State	Out of State	Total
Applicants	495	1,718	2,213
Interviewed	37	83	120
New students	8	16	24

FACTORS REQUIRED TO CONTINUE IN PROGRAM

3.5 overall and science GPA with no grade less than C

MCAT REQUIRED

Yes, minimum 9 in the verbal section and a 10 in each of the science sections or a total score of 31 with no sub-score less than 8

FINANCIAL AID

No special financial aid for students in the program

COST

	Resident Tuition and Fees ($)	Non Resident Tuition and Fees ($)
Undergraduate	43,800	43,800
Medical school	46,810	46,810

COLLEGE

Kean University

MEDICAL SCHOOL

Drexel University College of Medicine

ADDRESS

Office of Admission
Kean University
STEM Building, Suite 5-13
1000 Morris Avenue
Union, New Jersey 07083-7133
908-737-7200
http://njcste.kean.edu/programs/bsmd.html

NAME OF PROGRAM

4 + 4 Bachelor of Science/Medical Degree (BS/MD)
Scholars Program

LENGTH OF PROGRAM

8 years

APPLICATION DEADLINE

December 1

INFORMATION ABOUT THE PROGRAM

Students have an integrated program of biology, chemistry, physics, and math during their freshman and sophomore years. The final two years involve a concentration in biomedical sciences, including a preceptorship in which they shadow physicians at St. Peter's University Hospital in New Brunswick, New Jersey. Students earn a bachelor of science in science and technology/biomedicine.

Medical students return to St. Peter's University Hospital for at least one third-year clerkship and one fourth-year rotation.

TRANSFER STUDENTS CONSIDERED

No

CITIZENSHIP REQUIREMENTS

U.S. citizen or permanent resident visa

MINIMUM REQUIRED FACTORS IN SELECTION

CLASSES

Four years of math and English, three years of science including at least one semester each of biology, chemistry and physics.

GPA

3.5 unweighted GPA

SAT

1,270 critical reading and math, with no sub-score lower than 560.

ACT

28

2010–2011 ACCEPTANCES

	In State	Out of State	Total
Applicants			
Interviewed			
New students			

No information provided

FACTORS REQUIRED TO CONTINUE IN PROGRAM

3.5 overall and science GPA

MCAT REQUIRED

Yes, minimum 9 in the verbal section and a 10 in each of the science sections

FINANCIAL AID

No special financial aid for students in the program

COST

	Resident Tuition and Fees ($)	Non Resident Tuition and Fees ($)
Undergraduate	17,300	22,765
Medical school	46,810	46,810

COLLEGE
Lehigh University

MEDICAL SCHOOL
Drexel University College of Medicine

ADDRESS
Office of Admissions
Lehigh University
27 Memorial Drive West
Bethlehem, Pennsylvania 18015-3027
610-758-3100
www.lehigh.edu/~inbios/ugrad/combined.htm

NAME OF PROGRAM
Combined Degree Program in Medicine

LENGTH OF PROGRAM
7 years

APPLICATION DEADLINE
November 15

INFORMATION ABOUT THE PROGRAM
Students may major in any subject at Lehigh, although there are
a number of required courses for the program, so careful planning
is required.

TRANSFER STUDENTS CONSIDERED
No

CITIZENSHIP REQUIREMENTS
U.S. citizen or permanent resident visa

MINIMUM REQUIRED FACTORS IN SELECTION

CLASSES

No specific requirement

GPA

Top five percent of high school class; recently accepted students had an average 3.7 unweighted GPA.

SAT

1,360 critical reading and math; recently accepted students had on average 720 critical reading score and a 780 math score; Subject tests highly recommended—math level 1 or 2 and chemistry.

ACT

31

2011–2012 ACCEPTANCES

	In State	Out of State	Total
Applicants	30	183	213
Interviewed	4	25	29
New students	0	0	0

FACTORS REQUIRED TO CONTINUE IN PROGRAM

3.5 overall and science and math GPA with no grade less than a C

MCAT REQUIRED

Yes; minimum score of 9 on verbal section and 10 on each of the science sections; alternatively, a combined score of 31 with no subscore below 8

FINANCIAL AID

No special financial aid for students in the program

COST

	Resident Tuition and Fees ($)	Non Resident Tuition and Fees ($)
Undergraduate	42,220	42,220
Medical school	46,810	46,810

COLLEGE
Monmouth University

MEDICAL SCHOOL
Drexel University College of Medicine

ADDRESS
Office of Undergraduate Admission
Monmouth University
400 Cedar Avenue
West Long Branch, New Jersey 07764-1898
732-571-3456
www.monmouth.edu/academics/pre-professional_health
/medical_scholars.asp

NAME OF PROGRAM
Monmouth Medical Center Scholars Program

LENGTH OF PROGRAM
8 years

APPLICATION DEADLINE
December 1

INFORMATION ABOUT THE PROGRAM
The focus of this program is on training students who wish to enter family medicine, internal medicine, or pediatrics. Students participate in health-related activities at Monmouth Medical Center, including experience in clinical medicine. The program also provides career counseling, MCAT preparation, and practice interviews. There are two applications for this program, one to Monmouth University and a Drexel University supplemental application.

TRANSFER STUDENTS CONSIDERED
No

CITIZENSHIP REQUIREMENTS
U.S. citizen or permanent resident visa; New Jersey residents only

MINIMUM REQUIRED FACTORS IN SELECTION

CLASSES

No specific requirement

GPA

3.5 unweighted

SAT

1,270 critical reading and math, with no sub-score lower than 560

ACT

28

2010–2011 ACCEPTANCES

	In State	Out of State	Total
Applicants			
Interviewed			
New students			

No information provided

FACTORS REQUIRED TO CONTINUE IN PROGRAM

3.5 overall and science GPA with no grade less than a C in any class

MCAT REQUIRED

Yes; minimum score of 10 on biological and physical science sections and 9 on verbal section; alternatively, a minimum total score of 31 with no subsection score less than 8.

FINANCIAL AID

No special financial aid for students in the program

COST

	Resident Tuition and Fees ($)	Non Resident Tuition and Fees ($)
Undergraduate	30,041	not applicable
Medical school	46,810	not applicable

COLLEGE
Muhlenberg College *affiliated c̄ Evangelical Lutheran church in America*

MEDICAL SCHOOL
Drexel University College of Medicine

ADDRESS
Coordinator of 4-4 Program
Office of Admission
Muhlenberg College
2400 Chew Street
Allentown, Pennsylvania 18104-5586
484-664-3200
www.muhlenberg.edu/main/admissions/Drexel4-4.html

NAME OF PROGRAM
4-4 Early Assurance Program

LENGTH OF PROGRAM
8 years

APPLICATION DEADLINE
January 1

INFORMATION ABOUT THE PROGRAM
Personal interviews with Muhlenberg are required and must be completed by the January 1 deadline.

TRANSFER STUDENTS CONSIDERED
No

CITIZENSHIP REQUIREMENTS
U.S. citizen or permanent resident visa; Canadian residents also considered. Preference given to students who reside in the Middle Atlantic Region of Pennsylvania, New Jersey, New York, Delaware or Maryland.

MINIMUM REQUIRED FACTORS IN SELECTION

CLASSES

No specific requirement

GPA

No specific requirements; successful students are normally in the top five percent of their high school class.

SAT

1,270 critical reading and math with no sub-score less than 560; Successful students normally score 1,300 or higher on the critical reading and math. The average unweighted GPA was 3.65.

ACT

28

2010–2011 ACCEPTANCES

	In State	Out of State	Total
Applicants	6	43	49
Interviewed	3	12	15
New students	2	9	11

FACTORS REQUIRED TO CONTINUE IN PROGRAM

3.5 overall and science GPA

MCAT REQUIRED

Yes. Minimum score of 10 on the biological and physical science sections and a 9 on the verbal section

FINANCIAL AID

No special financial aid for students in the program

COST

	Resident Tuition and Fees ($)	Non Resident Tuition and Fees ($)
Undergraduate	41,510	41,510
Medical school	46,810	46,810

COLLEGE
Robert Morris University

MEDICAL SCHOOL
Drexel University College of Medicine

ADDRESS
Robert Morris University
6001 University Boulevard
Moon Township, Pennsylvania 15108-2574
800-762-0097
http://sentry.rmu.edu/web/cms/schools/sems/science/pre-med/
Pages/drexel.aspx

NAME OF PROGRAM
Scholars Articulation Program

LENGTH OF PROGRAM
8 years

APPLICATION DEADLINE
No information provided

INFORMATION ABOUT THE PROGRAM
This program is a collaboration between Robert Morris University, Drexel University College of Medicine, and Allegheny General Hospital. As undergraduates, students participate in a research course at Allegheny General Hospital. Preference in admissions is given to students interested in family medicine, general internal medicine, and general pediatrics.

TRANSFER STUDENTS CONSIDERED
No

CITIZENSHIP REQUIREMENTS
U.S. citizen or permanent resident visa; preference given to residents of Ohio, Pennsylvania and West Virginia.

MINIMUM REQUIRED FACTORS IN SELECTION

CLASSES

No specific requirements

GPA

3.5 unweighted

SAT

1,270 critical reading and math

ACT

24

2010–2011 ACCEPTANCES

	In State	Out of State	Total
Applicants			
Interviewed			
New students			

No information provided

FACTORS REQUIRED TO CONTINUE IN PROGRAM

Overall and science GPA of 3.5

MCAT REQUIRED

Yes; minimum 31

FINANCIAL AID

No special financial aid for students in the program

COST

	Resident Tuition and Fees ($)	Non Resident Tuition and Fees ($)
Undergraduate	24,020	24,020
Medical school	46,810	46,810

COLLEGE
Rosemont College

MEDICAL SCHOOL
Drexel University College of Medicine

ADDRESS
Rosemont College
Office of Admissions
1400 Montgomery Avenue
Rosemont, Pennsylvania 19010-1631
610-526-2966
www.rosemont.edu/uc/special-programs-dual-degrees/

NAME OF PROGRAM
Early Assurance Program/Fast Track Program

LENGTH OF PROGRAM
7 or 8 years

APPLICATION DEADLINE
December 1

INFORMATION ABOUT THE PROGRAM
Rosemont has two programs with Drexel. The Early Assurance Program is an eight-year program. The Fast Track Program is a seven-year program. Students are required to interview at Rosemont as well as Drexel. Students who meet the minimum requirements for the program will receive a Drexel College of Medicine supplemental application, which must be submitted by January 1.

TRANSFER STUDENTS CONSIDERED
No

CITIZENSHIP REQUIREMENTS
U.S. citizen or permanent resident visa

MINIMUM REQUIRED FACTORS IN SELECTION

CLASSES

Full academic course load including three years of foreign language for Early Assurance Program, four years of English and math, as well as at least one semester each of biology, chemistry, and physics.

GPA

Top ten percent of high school class and 3.5 unweighted GPA

SAT

1,300 critical reading and math with no sub-score below 600 for the Early Assurance Program; 1,360 critical reading and math with no sub-score below 560 for the Fast Track Program; writing score is not considered.

ACT

31 for Fast Track Program. 29 for Early Assurance Program

2010–2011 ACCEPTANCES

	In State	Out of State	Total
Applicants			11 Fast 15 Early
Interviewed			3 Fast 6 Early
New students			2 Fast 1 Early

FACTORS REQUIRED TO CONTINUE IN PROGRAM

3.5 GPA and 3.25 science GPA

MCAT REQUIRED

Yes, minimum score of 31

FINANCIAL AID

No special financial aid for students in the program

COST

	Resident Tuition and Fees ($)	Non Resident Tuition and Fees ($)
Undergraduate	29,500	29,500
Medical school	46,810	46,810

COLLEGE
Ursinus College

MEDICAL SCHOOL
Drexel University College of Medicine

ADDRESS
Ursinus College
Office of Admission
601 E. Main Street
Collegeville, Pennsylvania 19426-1000
610-409-3000
www.ursinus.edu/netcommunity/page.aspx?pid=440

NAME OF PROGRAM
Early Assurance Program

LENGTH OF PROGRAM
8 years

APPLICATION DEADLINE
November 15

INFORMATION ABOUT THE PROGRAM
Top candidates for the program are chosen in December and then
sent additional information about the program. These candidates
are interviewed by the undergraduate college in January, and decisions are made on who to recommend to the medical school. The
medical school will decide who to interview in February.

TRANSFER STUDENTS CONSIDERED
No

CITIZENSHIP REQUIREMENTS
U.S. citizen or permanent resident visa; must be a graduate of a
U.S. high school

MINIMUM REQUIRED FACTORS IN SELECTION

CLASSES

Four years of English and math, three years of science including one year each of biology, chemistry and physics

GPA

Top ten percent of high school class

SAT

1,300 critical reading and math with no sub-score below 560; writing score is not considered.

ACT

No specific requirement

2010–2011 ACCEPTANCES

	In State	Out of State	Total
Applicants			
Interviewed			
New students			

No information provided

FACTORS REQUIRED TO CONTINUE IN PROGRAM

3.5 overall and science GPA with no grade less than a C in any class

MCAT REQUIRED

Yes, minimum score of 10 on biological and physical science sections and 9 on verbal section. Alternatively, a minimum total score of 31 with no subsection score less than 8

FINANCIAL AID

No special financial aid for students in the program

COST

	Resident Tuition and Fees ($)	Non Resident Tuition and Fees ($)
Undergraduate	43,100	43,100
Medical school	46,810	46,810

COLLEGE
Villanova University

MEDICAL SCHOOL
Drexel University College of Medicine

ADDRESS
Health Professions Advisor
Villanova University
800 Lancaster Avenue
Villanova, Pennsylvania 19085-1603
610-519-6000
www1.villanova.edu/villanova/artsci/undergrad/health.html
/affiliates/medicine.html

NAME OF PROGRAM
Medical Affiliate Program

LENGTH OF PROGRAM
7 years

APPLICATION DEADLINE
November 1

INFORMATION ABOUT THE PROGRAM
Students may major in any major offered by Villanova, although
some majors are more difficult to complete in the three years the
student is at the college. The most common major is biology, followed by comprehensive science. Students who meet the basic requirements will be asked to submit a supplemental application to
the medical school.

TRANSFER STUDENTS CONSIDERED
No

CITIZENSHIP REQUIREMENTS
U.S. citizen or permanent resident visa; must be a graduate of a
U.S. high school

MINIMUM REQUIRED FACTORS IN SELECTION

CLASSES

Four years of math, four years of English, three years of science including at least one semester each of biology, chemistry, and physics

GPA

Top five percent of class; 3.8 unweighted; average GPA for admitted students was 3.90 unweighted

SAT

1,360 critical reading and math with no sub-score below 600; SAT subject tests recommended but not required

ACT

31 plus writing

2011–2012 ACCEPTANCES

	In State	Out of State	Total
Applicants	75	414	489
Interviewed	9	45	54
New students	1	10	11

FACTORS REQUIRED TO CONTINUE IN PROGRAM

Students must maintain a 3.5 overall and science GPA; no grade less than a C

MCAT REQUIRED

Yes, with minimum score of 9 on verbal reasoning, 10 in physical sciences, and 10 in biological sciences or a combined score of 31 with no sub-score less than 8.

FINANCIAL AID

No special financial aid for students in the program

COST

	Resident Tuition and Fees ($)	Non Resident Tuition and Fees ($)
Undergraduate	42,740	42,740
Medical school	46,810	46,810

COLLEGE
West Chester University

MEDICAL SCHOOL
Drexel University College of Medicine

ADDRESS
West Chester University of Pennsylvania
700 South High Street
West Chester, Pennsylvania 19383-0001
610-436-1000
www.wcupa.edu/_ACADEMICS/SCH_CAS/MED/Early_
Assurance_Undergrad/drexel.asp

NAME OF PROGRAM
Pre-Medical Program

LENGTH OF PROGRAM
8 years

APPLICATION DEADLINE
November 15

INFORMATION ABOUT THE PROGRAM
Students must submit an application to the college and a supplemental application to Drexel College of Medicine. Students must have documented health care experience.

TRANSFER STUDENTS CONSIDERED
No

CITIZENSHIP REQUIREMENTS
U.S. citizen or permanent resident visa

MINIMUM REQUIRED FACTORS IN SELECTION

CLASSES

Four years of English and math, three years of science including one year each of biology, chemistry and physics

GPA

Top ten percent of high school class and unweighted GPA of 3.5

SAT

1,300 critical reading and math, with no sub-score lower than 560

ACT

No specific requirement

2010–2011 ACCEPTANCES

	In State	Out of State	Total
Applicants			
Interviewed			
New students			

No information provided

FACTORS REQUIRED TO CONTINUE IN PROGRAM

3.5 overall and science GPA with no grade lower than C in any course

MCAT REQUIRED

Yes, with minimum score of 9 on verbal reasoning, 10 in physical sciences, and 10 in biological sciences, or a combined score of 31 with no sub-score less than 8

FINANCIAL AID

No special financial aid for students in the program

COST

	Resident Tuition and Fees ($)	Non Resident Tuition and Fees ($)
Undergraduate	8,620	18,446
Medical school	46,810	46,810

COLLEGE

Penn State University

MEDICAL SCHOOL

Jefferson Medical College

ADDRESS

Penn State University
Eberly College of Science
Undergraduate Recruitment Office
108 Whitmore Laboratory
University Park, Pennsylvania 16802-1014
814-865-2609
www.science.psu.edu/premed/premedmed
/accelerated-premed-medical/

NAME OF PROGRAM

Penn State's Accelerated Premedical-Medical Program

LENGTH OF PROGRAM

6 or 7 years

APPLICATION DEADLINE

November 30

INFORMATION ABOUT THE PROGRAM

Students can choose either a six-year or seven-year program. The six-year program requires students to spend two years plus two summers at Penn State before entering Jefferson Medical College for four years. Students choosing the seven-year program spend three years at Penn State, no summers required, followed by four years at Jefferson.

Non-academic factors considered include motivation, compassion, integrity, and dedication.

TRANSFER STUDENTS CONSIDERED

No

CITIZENSHIP REQUIREMENTS
International students considered; preference given to qualified residents of Pennsylvania

MINIMUM REQUIRED FACTORS IN SELECTION

CLASSES

Four years of English, three years of math, three years of science, and five years of social studies, humanities, or arts.

GPA

Top ten percent of high school class

SAT

2,100 from a single test date; average test score for class entering 2011 was 2,260

ACT

32

2011–2012 ACCEPTANCES

	In State	Out of State	Total
Applicants	98	551	649
Interviewed	23	73	96
New students	9	21	30

FACTORS REQUIRED TO CONTINUE IN PROGRAM

3.5 overall and science GPA

MCAT REQUIRED

Yes; average score of 9 or better on each section of the MCAT and a composite score of at least 30

FINANCIAL AID

Students not eligible for tuition scholarships from Schreyer Honors College or Braddock Scholarships from the Eberly College of Science

COST

	Resident Tuition and Fees ($)	Non Resident Tuition and Fees ($)
Undergraduate	15,562	27,864
Medical school	50,936	50,936

COLLEGE

Wilkes University

MEDICAL SCHOOL

Penn State Hershey College of Medicine

ADDRESS

Wilkes University
84 West South Street
Wilkes-Barre, Pennsylvania 18766-0003
800-945-5378
www.wilkes.edu/pages/424.asp

NAME OF PROGRAM

Guthrie or WVHCS Premedical Scholars Program

LENGTH OF PROGRAM

8 years

APPLICATION DEADLINE

November 15

INFORMATION ABOUT THE PROGRAM

Students must be committed to a career in family practice
medicine.

TRANSFER STUDENTS CONSIDERED

No

CITIZENSHIP REQUIREMENTS

U.S. citizen or permanent resident visa; must be from a rural or
medically underserved area of Pennsylvania

MINIMUM REQUIRED FACTORS IN SELECTION

CLASSES

No specific requirement

GPA

Top ten percent of high school class

SAT

1,250 critical reading and math

ACT

No specific requirement

2010–2011 ACCEPTANCES

	In State	Out of State	Total
Applicants	0		
Interviewed	0		
New students	0		0

No other information provided

FACTORS REQUIRED TO CONTINUE IN PROGRAM

3.5 overall and science GPA

MCAT REQUIRED

Yes; minimum score equal to previous year's average of incoming class; for 2010 that score was a 30 with no sub-score below 9

FINANCIAL AID

No special financial aid for students in the program.

COST

	Resident Tuition and Fees ($)	Non Resident Tuition and Fees ($)
Undergraduate	29,326	not applicable
Medical school	42,542	not applicable

COLLEGE
Duquesne University

MEDICAL SCHOOL
Temple University School of Medicine

ADDRESS
Duquesne University
Office of Admission
600 Forbes Avenue
Pittsburgh, Pennsylvania 15282-0001
412-396-6222
www.duq.edu/academics/degrees-and-programs/pre-med
/pre-med-affiliations

NAME OF PROGRAM
Medical Scholars Program

LENGTH OF PROGRAM
8 years

APPLICATION DEADLINE
November 15 for Duquesne

INFORMATION ABOUT THE PROGRAM
Duquesne interviews students before deciding which students to
recommend to Temple. Temple also interviews students in whom
they have an interest. Students may major in any subject as long
as the premedical science requirements are met.

TRANSFER STUDENTS CONSIDERED
No

CITIZENSHIP REQUIREMENTS
U.S. citizen or permanent resident visa

MINIMUM REQUIRED FACTORS IN SELECTION

CLASSES

No specific requirement. AP coursework is expected.

GPA

Top five percent of the student's high school class

SAT

1,350 critical reading and math; no section under 600, including writing

ACT

31

2011–2012 ACCEPTANCES

	In State	Out of State	Total
Applicants	37		37
Interviewed	15		15
New students	11		11

Note: these numbers reflect applications and admissions for all three programs associated with Temple University School of Medicine.

FACTORS REQUIRED TO CONTINUE IN PROGRAM

3.5 overall and science GPA with no grade less than C during the first three years of undergraduate study. The minimum GPA for the fourth year of undergraduate study is a 3.0,with no grade less than C.

MCAT REQUIRED

Yes; minimum 30 with no less than 8 on any section

FINANCIAL AID

No special financial aid for students in the program

COST

	Resident Tuition and Fees ($)	Non Resident Tuition and Fees ($)
Undergraduate	27,668	27,668
Medical school	44,244	54,058

COLLEGE
Washington & Jefferson College

MEDICAL SCHOOL
Temple University School of Medicine

ADDRESS
Washington & Jefferson College
Office of Admission
60 South Lincoln Street
Washington, Pennsylvania 15301-4812
724-223-6025
www.washjeff.edu/pre-health-program
/health-professions-school-affiliations

NAME OF PROGRAM
Medical Scholars Program

LENGTH OF PROGRAM
8 years

APPLICATION DEADLINE
As early in the fall as possible for Washington & Jefferson; January 1 for the Medical Scholars Program

INFORMATION ABOUT THE PROGRAM
Students first apply to Washington & Jefferson and after being accepted apply to the Medical Scholars Program. Washington & Jefferson interviews students before deciding which students to recommend to Temple. Temple also interviews students in whom they have an interest. Students may apply to other medical schools but will lose their guaranteed seat if they do so.

TRANSFER STUDENTS CONSIDERED
No

CITIZENSHIP REQUIREMENTS
U.S. citizen or permanent resident visa.

MINIMUM REQUIRED FACTORS IN SELECTION

CLASSES

No specific requirement although AP science coursework is expected.

GPA

Top five percent of the student's high school class

SAT

1,350 critical reading and math; no section under 600, including writing

ACT

31

2011–2012 ACCEPTANCES

	In State	Out of State	Total
Applicants	37		37
Interviewed	15		15
New students	11		11

Note: these numbers reflect applications and admissions for all three programs associated with Temple University School of Medicine.

FACTORS REQUIRED TO CONTINUE IN PROGRAM

3.5 science GPA with no grade less than a C

MCAT REQUIRED

Yes; minimum 30 with no less than 8 on any section

FINANCIAL AID

No special financial aid for students in the program

COST

	Resident Tuition and Fees ($)	Non Resident Tuition and Fees ($)
Undergraduate	38,310	38,310
Medical school	44,244	54,058

COLLEGE
Widener University

MEDICAL SCHOOL
Temple University School of Medicine

ADDRESS
Health Professions Advisor
Widener University
One University Place
Chester, Pennsylvania 19013-5700
610-499-4030
www.widener.edu/academics/schools/arts_sciences/sciences
/premed/medical_scholars.aspx

NAME OF PROGRAM
Medical Scholars Program

LENGTH OF PROGRAM
8 years

APPLICATION DEADLINE
December 15 for Widener; January 1 for Temple

INFORMATION ABOUT THE PROGRAM
Widener interviews students before deciding which students to recommend to Temple. Temple also interviews students in whom they have an interest. Students may major in any subject.

TRANSFER STUDENTS CONSIDERED
No

CITIZENSHIP REQUIREMENTS
U.S. citizen or permanent resident visa; students in the Widener program must be from Pennsylvania, Delaware, New Jersey, or Maryland and have an interest in family medicine, general internal medicine, or general pediatrics.

MINIMUM REQUIRED FACTORS IN SELECTION

CLASSES

No specific requirement

GPA

Top five percent of the student's high school class

SAT

1,350 critical reading and math; no section under 600, including writing

ACT

31

2011–2012 ACCEPTANCES

	In State	Out of State	Total
Applicants	37		37
Interviewed	15		15
New students	11		11

Note: these numbers reflect applications and admissions for all three programs associated with Temple University School of Medicine.

FACTORS REQUIRED TO CONTINUE IN PROGRAM

3.5 GPA with no grade less than C during the first three years of undergraduate study. The minimum GPA for the fourth year of undergraduate study is a 3.0 with no grade less than C.

MCAT REQUIRED

Yes; minimum 30 with no less than 8 on any section

FINANCIAL AID

No special financial aid for students in the program

COST

	Resident Tuition and Fees ($)	Non Resident Tuition and Fees ($)
Undergraduate	36,382	36,382
Medical school	44,244	54,058

COLLEGE
University of Pittsburgh

MEDICAL SCHOOL
University of Pittsburgh School of Medicine

ADDRESS
University of Pittsburgh
Office of Admissions and Financial Aid
4227 Fifth Avenue
Alumni Hall
Pittsburgh, Pennsylvania 15260-6601
412-624-7488
www.medadmissions.pitt.edu/admissions-requirements
/guaranteed-admissions.php

NAME OF PROGRAM
Guaranteed admission

LENGTH OF PROGRAM
8 years

APPLICATION DEADLINE
December 1

INFORMATION ABOUT THE PROGRAM
Students interested in the program must indicate interest in pre-medicine or bioengineering on their undergraduate application. Students are required during the undergraduate years to continue medically related activities, including research and volunteer activities.

TRANSFER STUDENTS CONSIDERED
No

CITIZENSHIP REQUIREMENTS
U.S. citizen or permanent resident visa

MINIMUM REQUIRED FACTORS IN SELECTION

CLASSES

No specific requirement

GPA

No specific requirement

SAT

1,450 critical reading and math

ACT

33

2010–2011 ACCEPTANCES

	In State	Out of State	Total
Applicants			221
Interviewed			35
New students			8

FACTORS REQUIRED TO CONTINUE IN PROGRAM

3.75 overall and science GPA; must also engage in undergraduate research

MCAT REQUIRED

No, unless student wishes to be considered for merit scholarships or is applying to the MD/PhD program

FINANCIAL AID

No special financial aid for students in the program

COST

	Resident Tuition and Fees ($)	Non Resident Tuition and Fees ($)
Undergraduate	16,590	26,280
Medical school	45,509	46,629

COLLEGE

Inter American University of Puerto Rico at Ponce (UIA)

MEDICAL SCHOOL

Ponce School of Medicine

ADDRESS

Inter American University of Puerto Rico at Ponce
104 Turpo Industrial Park Road #1
Mercedita, PR 00715-1602
787-284-1912
www.psm.edu/Student_Affairs/Admissions/MD
/md_program_description.htm

NAME OF PROGRAM

Binary Programs

LENGTH OF PROGRAM

7 years

APPLICATION DEADLINE

December 15

INFORMATION ABOUT THE PROGRAM

The focus of the program is to educate physicians to provide medical care for Puerto Rico. In a recent class entering the medical
school, seventy-seven percent of the students came from Puerto
Rico and twenty-three percent from the continental U.S. Classes
are held in both English and Spanish, so students need to be proficient in Spanish.

TRANSFER STUDENTS CONSIDERED

No

CITIZENSHIP REQUIREMENTS

U.S. citizen or permanent resident visa; residents of Puerto Rico
are given preference

MINIMUM REQUIRED FACTORS IN SELECTION

None listed

2010–2011 ACCEPTANCES

	In State	Out of State	Total
Applicants			
Interviewed			
New students			

No information provided

FACTORS REQUIRED TO CONTINUE IN PROGRAM

Overall GPA of 3.2 and a 3.0 science GPA; must maintain minimum 3.0 GPA each semester

MCAT REQUIRED

Yes; minimum score of 20

FINANCIAL AID

No special financial aid for students in the program

COST

	Resident Tuition and Fees ($)	Non Resident Tuition and Fees ($)
Undergraduate	4,080	4,080
Medical school	26,308	39,220

COLLEGE

Pontifical Catholic University of Puerto Rico (PUCPR)

MEDICAL SCHOOL

Ponce School of Medicine

ADDRESS

Pontifical Catholic University of Puerto Rico
2250 Las Americas Avenue, Suite 284
Ponce, PR 00717-9777
787-841-2000
www.psm.edu/Student_Affairs/Admissions/MD
/md_program_description.htm

NAME OF PROGRAM

Binary Programs

LENGTH OF PROGRAM

6 years

APPLICATION DEADLINE

December 15

INFORMATION ABOUT THE PROGRAM

The focus of the program is to educate physicians to provide medical care for Puerto Rico. In a recent class entering the medical school, seventy-seven percent of the students came from Puerto Rico and twenty-three percent from the continental U.S. Classes are held in both English and Spanish, so students need to be proficient in Spanish.

TRANSFER STUDENTS CONSIDERED

No

CITIZENSHIP REQUIREMENTS

U.S. citizen or permanent resident visa; residents of Puerto Rico are given preference

MINIMUM REQUIRED FACTORS IN SELECTION

None listed

2010–2011 ACCEPTANCES

	In State	Out of State	Total
Applicants			
Interviewed			
New students			

No information provided

FACTORS REQUIRED TO CONTINUE IN PROGRAM

Overall GPA of 3.2 and a 3.0 science GPA; must maintain minimum 3.0 GPA each semester

MCAT REQUIRED

Yes; minimum score of 20

FINANCIAL AID

No special financial aid for students in the program

COST

	Resident Tuition and Fees ($)	Non Resident Tuition and Fees ($)
Undergraduate	5,318	5,318
Medical school	26,308	39,220

COLLEGE
Brown University

MEDICAL SCHOOL
Warren Alpert Medical School of Brown University

ADDRESS
PLME Office
Brown University
Biomedical Center 222
Box G-B222
Providence, Rhode Island 02912-0001
401-863-9790
www.brown.edu/academics/medical/plme/

NAME OF PROGRAM
Program in Liberal Medical Education (PLME)

LENGTH OF PROGRAM
8 years

APPLICATION DEADLINE
November 1 for early decision; January 1 for regular action

INFORMATION ABOUT THE PROGRAM
Brown University has no distribution requirements, and this carries over to the PLME. Students may study any of the almost one hundred majors available at Brown. PLME encourages students to pursue their interests in depth, whether in the natural sciences, the humanities, or the social sciences. Students may extend their undergraduate program by a year or two to pursue additional academic interests. Students may also work on an additional graduate degree such as a PhD or MPH while pursuing the BS/MD.

In addition to academics, PLME is looking for students who have motivation, maturity, character, and intellectual breadth.

PLME has enrichment activities including opportunities to observe physicians working, the chance to have an international experience while at Brown, and research opportunities.

PLME is unusual in that students can apply early decision to Brown and PLME. Students applying early decision have the opportunity to not attend Brown if they are not also admitted to PLME. Students accepted early decision to PLME will be informed of their admission in December.

PLME is also unusual in that interviews at the medical school are not required. Brown University does encourage students to have an interview with an alumni interviewer for the college. If students are admitted to Brown undergraduate, their application is considered by the PLME committee.

Students can apply to other medical schools, but in doing so they will lose their guaranteed spot at the medical school.

TRANSFER STUDENTS CONSIDERED

No

CITIZENSHIP REQUIREMENTS

International students considered

MINIMUM REQUIRED FACTORS IN SELECTION

CLASSES

Recommended are four years of English, three years of math, three years of foreign language, two years of science above freshman level, two years of history, and one year of coursework in elective academic subjects.

GPA

No minimum; eighty-eight percent of admitted students in top five percent of high school class and most are in the top 1%.

SAT

No minimum; average SAT scores over the last five years were critical reading, 725 to 738; math, 735 to 749; and writing 723 to 748; two subject tests required, one of which should be a science subject test

ACT

May be substituted for SAT and SAT subject tests; writing section required

2010–2011 ACCEPTANCES

	In State	Out of State	Total
Applicants	36	2,087	324 ED 1,697 Regular
Interviewed			
New students	6	49	17 ED 38 Regular

FACTORS REQUIRED TO CONTINUE IN PROGRAM

None listed

MCAT REQUIRED

No

FINANCIAL AID

Brown University meets one hundred percent of a student's financial need. Grants and loans are also available for the medical school.

COST

	Resident Tuition and Fees ($)	Non Resident Tuition and Fees ($)
Undergraduate	46,619	46,619
Medical school	51,137	51,137

COLLEGE
Fisk University

MEDICAL SCHOOL
Meharry Medical College

ADDRESS
Fisk University
1000 17th Avenue North
Nashville, Tennessee 37208-3045
615-329-8500
www.fisk.edu/Academics/PreProfessionalProgram
/PreProfessionalPreMedicine.aspx

NAME OF PROGRAM
Bachelor of Science/Doctor of Medicine Program

LENGTH OF PROGRAM
7 or 8 years

APPLICATION DEADLINE
February 1

INFORMATION ABOUT THE PROGRAM
Fisk is a historically black college, and the goal of this program is to train students underrepresented in the medical field. Students apply for this program while in high school, but the selection does not occur until after the first semester of college. Students are also expected to participate in a six-week academic and clinical enrichment program the summer after freshman year. Students accepted into the program can choose whether they are interested in a seven-year or eight-year program, as both are options. The most frequent major is biology, followed by chemistry.

TRANSFER STUDENTS CONSIDERED
No

CITIZENSHIP REQUIREMENTS
U.S. citizen or permanent resident visa

MINIMUM REQUIRED FACTORS IN SELECTION

CLASSES

No specific requirement

GPA

3.4 unweighted or top twenty percent of high school class, with a B or better in biology, chemistry, and advanced math courses

SAT

1,590

ACT

24

2011–2012 ACCEPTANCES

	In State	Out of State	Total
Applicants	3	3	6
Interviewed	2	2	4
New students	1	1	2

FACTORS REQUIRED TO CONTINUE IN PROGRAM

3.5 overall GPA

MCAT REQUIRED

Yes; minimum score of 24

FINANCIAL AID

Students in the program are given scholarships while enrolled at Fisk to cover the cost of their education.

COST

	Resident Tuition and Fees ($)	Non Resident Tuition and Fees ($)
Undergraduate	0	0
Medical school	48,426	48,426

COLLEGE
Grambling State University

MEDICAL SCHOOL
Meharry Medical College

ADDRESS
BS/MD Program Site Coordinator
Grambling State University
403 Main Street
Grambling, Louisiana 71245-2715
318-247-3811
www.gram.edu/academics/majors/arts%20and%20sciences
/departments/biology/training.php

NAME OF PROGRAM
Bachelor of Science/Doctor of Medicine Program

LENGTH OF PROGRAM
7 or 8 years

APPLICATION DEADLINE
Not provided

INFORMATION ABOUT THE PROGRAM
This program is designed to increase the number of African American physicians. Grambling and Meharry are both historically black colleges. Students may take seven or eight years to complete the program. Students must also agree to participate in a six-week summer program at the medical college designed to enrich the academic and clinic experiences.

TRANSFER STUDENTS CONSIDERED
No

CITIZENSHIP REQUIREMENTS
U.S. citizen or permanent resident visa

MINIMUM REQUIRED FACTORS IN SELECTION

CLASSES

No specific requirement

GPA

3.25 overall and science GPA

SAT

900 critical reading and math

ACT

20

2010–2011 ACCEPTANCES

	In State	Out of State	Total
Applicants			
Interviewed			
New students			

No information provided

FACTORS REQUIRED TO CONTINUE IN PROGRAM

None listed

MCAT REQUIRED

Not listed

FINANCIAL AID

Merit scholarships are available that may include full tuition.

COST

	Resident Tuition and Fees ($)	Non Resident Tuition and Fees ($)
Undergraduate	5,274	13,644
Medical school	48,426	48,426

COLLEGE
Baylor University

MEDICAL SCHOOL
Baylor College of Medicine

ADDRESS
Prehealth Studies Office
Baylor University
B.111 Baylor Science Building
One Bear Place #97341
Waco, Texas 76798-7341
254-710-3659
www.baylor.edu/prehealth/index.php?id=36430

NAME OF PROGRAM
Guaranteed Admission Program/Baylor2 Medical Track

LENGTH OF PROGRAM
8 years

APPLICATION DEADLINE
November 1

INFORMATION ABOUT THE PROGRAM
Four years of college at Baylor University are required as part of
the program. Students are encouraged to study abroad or work
on a research project if they have time during their four years at
Baylor University. According to Baylor University, the program
is designed to offer the best students the "opportunity to broaden
their educational horizons." Students should list pre-medicine as
their pre-professional area of study on the Baylor application. Students who meet the basic admissions criteria will be invited to
apply to the program.

Baylor University and Baylor College of Medicine are not affiliated institutions. Baylor College of Medicine is a private non-
sectarian institution.

TRANSFER STUDENTS CONSIDERED

No

CITIZENSHIP REQUIREMENTS

U.S. citizen or permanent resident visa

MINIMUM REQUIRED FACTORS IN SELECTION

CLASSES

No specific requirement

GPA

3.7 unweighted or top five percent of high school class

SAT

1,400 critical reading and math

ACT

32

2009–2010 ACCEPTANCES

	In State	Out of State	Total
Applicants			240
Interviewed			30
New students			6

FACTORS REQUIRED TO CONTINUE IN PROGRAM

3.4 overall GPA; 3.2 science GPA. Student receiving top scholarship has required GPA of 3.7. No grades lower than C. Must complete a modified application to Baylor College of Medicine.

MCAT REQUIRED

No

FINANCIAL AID

Grants, loans, and work study available for undergraduates. Limited financial aid for medical school.

COST

	Resident Tuition and Fees ($)	Non Resident Tuition and Fees ($)
Undergraduate	34,146	34,146
Medical school	15,618	28,768

COLLEGE

Rice University

MEDICAL SCHOOL

Baylor College of Medicine

ADDRESS

Rice University
Admission Office-MS 17
6100 South Main Street
Houston, Texas 77005-1827
713-348-7423
http://futureowls.rice.edu/futureowls
/Medical_Scholars_Program.asp

NAME OF PROGRAM

Medical Scholars Program

LENGTH OF PROGRAM

8 years

APPLICATION DEADLINE

December 1

INFORMATION ABOUT THE PROGRAM

"The Medical Scholars Program promotes the education of students who are scientifically competent, compassionate, and socially conscious." This is the stated goal of the program between Rice University and Baylor College of Medicine.

Students in this program are encouraged to explore all of the options available to Rice undergraduates. Explorations of the liberal arts and the student's own interests are also encouraged.

Students may apply to Rice regular decision or early decision. Those applying early decision must do so by the early decision date of November 1. If a student applies early decision and is admitted, they must commit to Rice by January 2 even though decisions by the Baylor College of Medicine will not be announced until late April. Rice will notify finalists in March, and Baylor conducts interviews in April. Students applying to the Rice/Baylor program may not apply to any of the other Baylor medical scholars programs.

The program is not binding, and students may apply out to other medical schools.

TRANSFER STUDENTS CONSIDERED

No

CITIZENSHIP REQUIREMENTS

International students considered

MINIMUM REQUIRED FACTORS IN SELECTION

CLASSES

NO SPECIFIC REQUIREMENT

GPA

No specific requirement; typical students in top five percent of high school class

SAT

No specific requirement; mid-range scores of students entering Rice, 1,350–1,510. Students must take two SAT subject tests, which should relate to your area of study.

ACT

No specific requirement, although SAT subject tests are not required if a student takes the ACT.

2011–2012 ACCEPTANCES

	In State	Out of State	Total
Applicants	145	213	358
Interviewed	14	13	27
New students	4	3	7

FACTORS REQUIRED TO CONTINUE IN PROGRAM

None listed

MCAT REQUIRED

No, unless the student is interested in the MD/PhD program.

FINANCIAL AID

Rice covers one hundred percent of a student's financial need. This makes available substantial financial aid to families with lower income levels. Like most medical schools, financial aid at Baylor is limited.

COST

	Resident Tuition and Fees ($)	Non Resident Tuition and Fees ($)
Undergraduate	37,292	37,292
Medical school	15,618	28,768

COLLEGE

University of Texas Pan American

MEDICAL SCHOOL

Baylor College of Medicine

ADDRESS

UTPA, Biology Department
1201 West University Drive
Edinburg, Texas 78539-2909
956-316-7025
http://portal.utpa.edu/utpa_main/daa_home/cose_home
/biology_home/biology_jp/jp_pmh

NAME OF PROGRAM

Premedical Honors College

LENGTH OF PROGRAM

8 years

APPLICATION DEADLINE

February 1

INFORMATION ABOUT THE PROGRAM

The goal of this program is to increase the number of physicians
serving the medically underserved area of South Texas. Students
are required to major in biology, chemistry, or biochemistry and
minor in one of the other sciences. Students complete two applications including one to the undergraduate college and one to the
premedical honors college.

TRANSFER STUDENTS CONSIDERED

No

CITIZENSHIP REQUIREMENTS

U.S. citizen or permanent resident visa; residence in South Texas

MINIMUM REQUIRED FACTORS IN SELECTION

CLASSES

No specific requirement

GPA

No specific requirement

SAT

No minimum score, but applicants must take the SAT

ACT

Not accepted.

2009–2010 ACCEPTANCES

	In State	Out of State	Total
Applicants	175		175
Interviewed			
New students	12		12

FACTORS REQUIRED TO CONTINUE IN PROGRAM

3.2 science GPA and 3.4 overall GPA

MCAT REQUIRED

Yes; minimum score 28 with no sub-score below 8

FINANCIAL AID

No special financial aid for students in the program

COST

	Resident Tuition and Fees ($)	Non Resident Tuition and Fees ($)
Undergraduate	6,124	not applicable
Medical school	15,618	not applicable

COLLEGE

Prairie View A & M University; South Texas College; Tarleton State University; Texas A & M International University; Texas A & M University at College Station; Texas A & M University at Commerce; Texas A & M University at Corpus Christi; Texas A & M University at Kingsville; West Texas A & M University

MEDICAL SCHOOL

Texas A & M Health Science Center College of Medicine

ADDRESS

Texas A&M Health Science Center College of Medicine
Office of Admissions
Partnership for Primary Care
8447 State Highway 47
Bryan, Texas 77807-3260
979-436-0233
http://medicine.tamhsc.edu/admissions/ppc/

NAME OF PROGRAM

Partnership for Primary Care

LENGTH OF PROGRAM

8 years

APPLICATION DEADLINE

1st Friday of February

INFORMATION ABOUT THE PROGRAM

This program is designed to help train students from rural areas of Texas that are facing a physician shortage. The focus of the program is training students in primary care medicine who will return to their home areas to practice medicine. Various medical enrichment activities are made available to students in the program, including workshops on success in medical school, medical seminars, and meetings with other students in the program.

There are also summer enrichment programs that students participate in as well as opportunities for doctor shadowing.

TRANSFER STUDENTS CONSIDERED

No

CITIZENSHIP REQUIREMENTS

U.S. citizen or permanent resident visa; resident of Texas; legal residence in a rural or underserved area or health professions shortage area as defined by the Health Professions Resource Center, Texas Department of Health

MINIMUM REQUIRED FACTORS IN SELECTION

CLASSES

No specific requirement

GPA

3.5 unweighted, and be predicted to graduate in top ten percent of high school class

SAT

1,200 on critical reading and math

ACT

26

2009–2010 ACCEPTANCES

	In State	Out of State	Total
Applicants			
Interviewed			
New students	15		15

No other information provided

FACTORS REQUIRED TO CONTINUE IN PROGRAM

3.25 GPA after freshman year and a 3.5 cumulative GPA in subsequent years; can have no grade in required courses below a C

MCAT REQUIRED

Yes; an MCAT score of at least 25 is required, with a minimum of 7 in any section.

FINANCIAL AID

No special financial aid for students in the program

COST

	Resident Tuition and Fees ($)	Non Resident Tuition and Fees ($)
Undergraduate	8,149	not applicable
Medical school	16,404	not applicable

COLLEGE
Texas Tech University

MEDICAL SCHOOL
Texas Tech University Health Sciences Center School of Medicine

ADDRESS
Texas Tech University Health Sciences Center
School of Medicine Office of Admissions 2B116
3601 4th Street MS 6216
Lubbock, Texas 79430-6216
806-743-2297
www.ttuhsc.edu/som/admissions/umsi.aspx

NAME OF PROGRAM
Undergraduate to Medical School Initiative

LENGTH OF PROGRAM
8 years

APPLICATION DEADLINE
December 1 for the application to the program

INFORMATION ABOUT THE PROGRAM
Students apply to the undergraduate college and the honors college and must be admitted before applying to the program. It takes four to six weeks for the undergraduate application to be processed, so students should plan on getting their undergraduate application submitted in early October. Must be a high school senior when applying to the program. Any study abroad program taken must be affiliated with Texas Tech University.

TRANSFER STUDENTS CONSIDERED
No

CITIZENSHIP REQUIREMENTS
U.S. citizen or permanent resident visa; Texas resident

MINIMUM REQUIRED FACTORS IN SELECTION

CLASSES

No specific requirements

GPA

3.70 unweighted; preference given to students ranking in the top ten percent of their class

SAT

1,300 critical reading and math

ACT

29

2010–2011 ACCEPTANCES

	In State	Out of State	Total
Applicants			
Interviewed			
New students			

No information provided

FACTORS REQUIRED TO CONTINUE IN PROGRAM

Science GPA of 3.6 and overall GPA of 3.7. A grade of B must be earned in all prerequisite courses.

MCAT REQUIRED

No

FINANCIAL AID

No special financial aid for students in the program

COST

	Resident Tuition and Fees ($)	Non Resident Tuition and Fees ($)
Undergraduate	8,942	not applicable
Medical school	14,417	not applicable

COLLEGE

The University of Texas at San Antonio

MEDICAL SCHOOL

The University of Texas Health Science Center at San Antonio

ADDRESS

The University of Texas at San Antonio
One UTSA Circle
San Antonio, Texas 78249-1644
210-458-4011
www.utsystem.edu/initiatives/time/fame.html

NAME OF PROGRAM

Facilitated Access to Medical Education (FAME)

LENGTH OF PROGRAM

7 years

APPLICATION DEADLINE

December 1, although the program recommends November 1.
Must be admitted to UTSA by December 1.

INFORMATION ABOUT THE PROGRAM

In response to the University of Texas System Request for Proposals to develop innovative and fully integrated pilot programs which lead to the award of both baccalaureate and Doctor of Medicine degrees, the University of Texas Health Science Center at San Antonio (UTHSCSA) and the University of Texas at San Antonio (UTSA) have partnered to implement an innovative program.

In order to meet degree requirements set for all college graduates in the State of Texas, core courses have been interwoven into a fully functional, collaborative seven- year curriculum with the end result of graduating physicians (Facilitated Acceptance to Medical Education [FAME] Program). This shared project uses traditional course structure, team-taught courses, and innovative seminar courses structured around disease-related experiences. The program was carefully developed to provide opportunities for students to exit the program should their interests take them to any number of other health-related fields. This program begins in Fall 2013.

Students must complete two applications including a University of Texas application and a FAME application.

TRANSFER STUDENTS CONSIDERED

No

CITIZENSHIP REQUIREMENTS
U.S. citizen or permanent resident visa; resident of Texas

MINIMUM REQUIRED FACTORS IN SELECTION

CLASSES
No specific requirement

GPA
3.6 science and overall GPA on a 4.0 scale or a 91 science and overall GPA on a 100 point scale

SAT
1,300 critical reading and math with minimum of 650 on each section

ACT
29 with a minimum of 29 on both the English and Math sections

2010–2011 ACCEPTANCES

	In State	Out of State	Total
Applicants			
Interviewed			
New students			

No information provided

FACTORS REQUIRED TO CONTINUE IN PROGRAM
3.6 overall and science GPA

MCAT REQUIRED
Yes. If the score is less than a 10 on the biological sciences section the student will need to take a biology enrichment course.

FINANCIAL AID
No special financial aid for students in the program

COST

	Resident Tuition and Fees ($)	Non Resident Tuition and Fees ($)
Undergraduate	8,660	not applicable
Medical school	17,115	not applicable

COLLEGE

The University of Texas at Dallas

MEDICAL SCHOOL

The University of Texas Southwestern Medical Center at Dallas

ADDRESS

Health Professions Advising Office
The University of Texas at Dallas
800 West Campbell Road
Richardson, Texas 75080-3021
972-883-2111
www.utdallas.edu/pre-health/ut-pact

NAME OF PROGRAM

UT-PACT BS/MD Program

LENGTH OF PROGRAM

7 years

APPLICATION DEADLINE

February 1

INFORMATION ABOUT THE PROGRAM

This is a pilot program as part of the initiative of the University of Texas to provide streamlined and better access to medical education to residents of Texas. Applicants are required to have a letter of recommendation from a high school guidance counselor and a high school math or science teacher and an additional letter of character reference, ideally from a health care professional. Students must be admitted to the undergraduate college by February 1; it takes about one month for applications to be processed. Early applications are encouraged. After admission to the college, students need to submit a secondary application to the program by February 15. Again, early applications are encouraged. Reference letters are due by February 15 also. Students will be notified of their status in the program by April 15.

TRANSFER STUDENTS CONSIDERED

No

CITIZENSHIP REQUIREMENTS

U.S. citizen or permanent resident visa; resident of Texas

MINIMUM REQUIRED FACTORS IN SELECTION

CLASSES

No specific requirement

GPA

3.5 unweighted GPA, average GPA of students attending the program is 3.88

SAT

Minimum 550 critical reading and 550 math; average SAT score of students attending the program is 1,487 critical reading and math.

ACT

27, average ACT of students attending the program is 28

2010–2011 ACCEPTANCES

	In State	Out of State	Total
Applicants			
Interviewed			
New students			

New program; no information exists for prior year

FACTORS REQUIRED TO CONTINUE IN PROGRAM

Overall and science GPA of 3.5

MCAT REQUIRED

No

FINANCIAL AID

No special financial aid for students in the program

COST

	Resident Tuition and Fees ($)	Non Resident Tuition and Fees ($)
Undergraduate	11,592	not applicable
Medical school	16,640	not applicable

COLLEGE

St. Mary's University; Texas A & M International University; University of Texas (UT) Pan American

MEDICAL SCHOOL

University of Texas Health Science Center at San Antonio

ADDRESS

Director of Admissions and Special Programs
School of Medicine
The University of Texas Health Science Center at San Antonio
7703 Floyd Curl Drive
San Antonio, Texas 78229-3900
210-567-6080
http://som.uthscsa.edu/Admissions
/earlyMatriculationProgram.asp

NAME OF PROGRAM

Facilitated Admissions for South Texas Scholars (FASTS)

LENGTH OF PROGRAM

8 years

APPLICATION DEADLINE

February 1

INFORMATION ABOUT THE PROGRAM

Students receive mentoring from medical school faculty as well as enrichment and clinical experiences in a Summer Premedical Academy. Students are expected to complete a biology or chemistry degree at one of the colleges. There is also an MCAT review course during the summer after junior year in college.

TRANSFER STUDENTS CONSIDERED

Yes

CITIZENSHIP REQUIREMENTS

U.S. citizen or permanent resident visa; Texas resident

MINIMUM REQUIRED FACTORS IN SELECTION

None listed

2010–2011 ACCEPTANCES

	In State	Out of State	Total
Applicants	24		24
Interviewed	14		14
New students	4		4

FACTORS REQUIRED TO CONTINUE IN PROGRAM

Overall and science GPA of 3.25 with no grade lower than a C

MCAT REQUIRED

Yes; ratio of GPA/MCAT will determine if student advances: students with ratio of 3.25/28, 3.5/26, 3.75/24, with no subsection score below a 7 are eligible for acceptance to the medical school.

FINANCIAL AID

No special financial aid for students in the program

COST

	Resident Tuition and Fees ($)	Non Resident Tuition and Fees ($)
Undergraduate	varies by college	not applicable
Medical school	17,115	not applicable

COLLEGE

Prairie View A & M University; Texas A & M International University; Texas Southern University; The University of Texas at Brownsville; The University of Texas at El Paso; The University of Texas-Pan American at Edinburg

MEDICAL SCHOOL

University of Texas Medical Branch at Galveston

ADDRESS

Director, Medical School Enrichment Programs
University of Texas Medical Branch
301 University Boulevard
Galveston, Texas 77555-0807
409-772-1212
www.utmb.edu/somstudentaffairs/specialprograms
/acceptanceprogram.html

NAME OF PROGRAM

Early Medical School Acceptance Program (EMSAP)

LENGTH OF PROGRAM

8 years

APPLICATION DEADLINE

January 31

INFORMATION ABOUT THE PROGRAM

Students participate in a summer enrichment program on the medical school campus that provides clinical exposure to the medical field. Students major in biology or chemistry. They will have continued clinical exposure during their four years of undergraduate study.

TRANSFER STUDENTS CONSIDERED

No

CITIZENSHIP REQUIREMENTS

U.S. citizen or permanent resident visa; Texas resident

MINIMUM REQUIRED FACTORS IN SELECTION

CLASSES

No specific requirement

GPA

High school average of 90 or above

SAT

1,200 on critical reading, math, and writing

ACT

20

2009–2010 ACCEPTANCES

	In State	Out of State	Total
Applicants			
Interviewed			
New students	30		30

No other information provided

FACTORS REQUIRED TO CONTINUE IN PROGRAM

3.25 GPA

MCAT REQUIRED

Yes; minimum score 24

FINANCIAL AID

No special financial aid for students in program

COST

	Resident Tuition and Fees ($)	Non Resident Tuition and Fees ($)
Undergraduate	varies by college	not applicable
Medical school	17,324	not applicable

COLLEGE

Virginia Commonwealth University

MEDICAL SCHOOL

Virginia Commonwealth University School of Medicine

ADDRESS

Virginia Commonwealth University
The Honors College
701 West Grace Street
Richmond, Virginia 23284-3010
804-828-1803
https://www.pubapps.vcu.edu/honors/guaranteed/medicine
/index.aspx

NAME OF PROGRAM

Guaranteed Admission Program (Medicine)

LENGTH OF PROGRAM

8 years

APPLICATION DEADLINE

November 15

INFORMATION ABOUT THE PROGRAM

Two applications are required for this program, an application for undergraduate admissions and an application for The Honors College Guaranteed Admission Program (Medicine). Students most commonly major in biology or chemistry, although other majors are possible. There are a number of required science courses for this program, so other majors require careful planning. Students must complete 120 hours of health care related experience each year during the first three years of the program and sixty additional hours the fourth year. During the third year of the program, students complete a one-semester mentorship with a faculty member of the medical school. Accepted students have an average of 450 hours of health care related experience.

TRANSFER STUDENTS CONSIDERED

No

CITIZENSHIP REQUIREMENTS

U.S. citizen or permanent resident visa; Canadian residents also considered; preference is given to Virginia residents.

MINIMUM REQUIRED FACTORS IN SELECTION

CLASSES

Four years of English, three years of math, three years of science, and three years of history or social studies; three years of a foreign language are strongly encouraged.

GPA

3.5 unweighted; average GPA of accepted students, 3.87 unweighted

SAT

1,910 with no sub-score below 530; average SAT score of accepted students, 2,120.

ACT

29; note that SAT is preferred but the ACT will be accepted.

2010–2011 ACCEPTANCES

	In State	Out of State	Total
Applicants	85	136	221
Interviewed	26	34	60
New students	13	9	22

FACTORS REQUIRED TO CONTINUE IN PROGRAM

Cumulative and science GPA of 3.5

MCAT REQUIRED

No

FINANCIAL AID

No special financial aid for students in the program

COST

	Resident Tuition and Fees ($)	Non Resident Tuition and Fees ($)
Undergraduate	9,886	23,912
Medical school	30,460	45,418

COLLEGE
Shepherd University

MEDICAL SCHOOL
West Virginia School of Medicine

ADDRESS
Shepherd University
P.O. Box 3210
Shepherdstown, West Virginia 25443-3210
304-876-5227
www.shepherd.edu/university/medstep/

NAME OF PROGRAM
MedSTEP

LENGTH OF PROGRAM
8 years

APPLICATION DEADLINE
No information provided

INFORMATION ABOUT THE PROGRAM
Most students will major in biology or chemistry. The focus of the program is on increasing the number of physicians in the Eastern Panhandle of West Virginia.

TRANSFER STUDENTS CONSIDERED
No

CITIZENSHIP REQUIREMENTS
U.S. citizen or permanent resident visa

MINIMUM REQUIRED FACTORS IN SELECTION

CLASSES

No specific requirements

GPA

3.75 unweighted

SAT

1,100

ACT

24

2010–2011 ACCEPTANCES

	In State	Out of State	Total
Applicants			
Interviewed			
New students			

No information provided

FACTORS REQUIRED TO CONTINUE IN PROGRAM

Science GPA of 3.5

MCAT REQUIRED

Yes; must score at or above the minimum score required for admission to the West Virginia University School of Medicine.

FINANCIAL AID

No special financial aid for students in the program

COST

	Resident Tuition and Fees ($)	Non Resident Tuition and Fees ($)
Undergraduate	5,834	15,136
Medical school	23,493	50,181

COLLEGE
Caldwell College

MEDICAL SCHOOL
St. George's University School of Medicine—
Grenada, West Indies

ADDRESS
Caldwell College
120 Bloomfield Avenue
Caldwell, New Jersey 07006-5310
973-618-3000
www.caldwell.edu/health-professionals/Affiliation.aspx

NAME OF PROGRAM
Health Professions Affiliation Program Medicine

LENGTH OF PROGRAM
7 or 8 years

APPLICATION DEADLINE
January 15

INFORMATION ABOUT THE PROGRAM
Students can major in any topic.

TRANSFER STUDENTS CONSIDERED
No

CITIZENSHIP REQUIREMENTS
U.S. citizen or permanent resident visa

MINIMUM REQUIRED FACTORS IN SELECTION

CLASSES
No specific requirements

GPA
3.5 unweighted

SAT
1,200 critical reading and math

ACT
26

2010–2011 ACCEPTANCES

	In State	Out of State	Total
Applicants			
Interviewed			
New students			

No information provided

FACTORS REQUIRED TO CONTINUE IN PROGRAM
No information provided

MCAT REQUIRED
No information provided.

FINANCIAL AID
No special financial aid for students in the program

COST

	Resident Tuition and Fees ($)	Non Resident Tuition and Fees ($)
Undergraduate	28,185	28,185
Medical school	23,759	23,759

COLLEGE
New Jersey Institute of Technology

MEDICAL SCHOOL
St. George's University School of Medicine—
Grenada, West Indies

ADDRESS
Honors College
New Jersey Institute of Technology
University Heights
Newark, New Jersey 07102-1982
973-642-7664
http://honors.njit.edu/admission/pre-health-law/health.php

NAME OF PROGRAM
Accelerated Medical Program

LENGTH OF PROGRAM
7 years

APPLICATION DEADLINE
November 1

INFORMATION ABOUT THE PROGRAM
Students spend their first three years at the New Jersey Institute
of Technology, the next two years in Grenada and the final two
years at St. Michael's Medical Center adjoining NJIT.

TRANSFER STUDENTS CONSIDERED
No

CITIZENSHIP REQUIREMENTS
U.S. citizen or permanent resident visa

MINIMUM REQUIRED FACTORS IN SELECTION

CLASSES

No specific requirements

GPA

Top 10%

SAT

1,300

ACT

30

2010–2011 ACCEPTANCES

	In State	Out of State	Total
Applicants			
Interviewed			
New students			

No information provided

FACTORS REQUIRED TO CONTINUE IN PROGRAM

No information provided

MCAT REQUIRED

Yes; test results do not affect admissions.

FINANCIAL AID

No special financial aid for students in the program

COST

	Resident Tuition and Fees ($)	Non Resident Tuition and Fees ($)
Undergraduate	14,740	27,040
Medical school	23,759	23,759

Index

For over a decade Todd Johnson has provided college admissions counseling to students throughout the United States. He has helped hundreds of students become the strongest candidates for BS/MD programs.

Todd is a graduate of St. Olaf College and the law school at Washington University in St. Louis, where he was the executive editor of the law review. Todd can be reached through his company website, www.collegeadmissionspartners.com.